D1345473

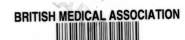

Surgical Treatment of Hemorrhoids

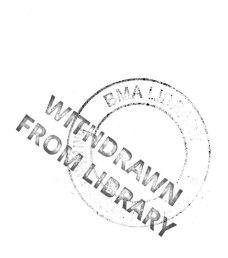

Indru Khubchandani Nina Paonessa
and Khawaja Azimuddin (Eds.)

Surgical Treatment of Hemorrhoids

Second Edition

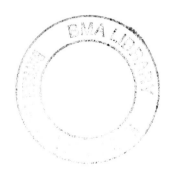

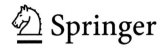

Editors

Indru Khubchandani, MD, FACS, FRCS
Professor of Surgery
Penn State University at Hershey
Adjunct Professor of Surgery
Drexel University at Hahnemann
Philadelphia
Division of Colon and Rectal Surgery
Allentown, PA, USA
IndruK@aol.com

Nina Paonessa, DO, FACOS
Clinical Assistant Professor of Surgery
Penn State University at Hershey
Division of Colon and Rectal Surgery
Allentown, PA, USA
npaonessa@yahoo.com

Khawaja Azimuddin, DO, FACOS
Houston, TX, USA
kazimuddin@hotmail.com

ISBN 978-1-84800-313-2   e-ISBN 978-1-84800-314-9
DOI 10.1007/978-1-84800-314-9

British Library Cataloguing in Publication Data
A catalogue record for this book is available from the British Library

Library of Congress Control Number: 2008939377

Printed on acid-free paper

Springer Science+Business Media
springer.com

*Dedicated to our patients, who have provided
the inspiration for this work*

Foreword

It is a great honor to be asked to contribute a Foreword in recognition of a peer's contribution to the literature in the field of colon and rectal surgery, and a special privilege to be asked by someone who is inarguably as recognized an international authority as Indru Khubchandani—as well as his colleagues. I have known Dr. Khubchandani for more than thirty years. He was born in Bombay, India, and attended college and medical school in that city, achieving his M.D. degree in 1956. From there he traveled to Sunderland, England, where he became a House Officer, ultimately moving to Ryhope in order to complete his training as a senior registrar. He became a Fellow of the Royal College of Surgeons of England and Edinburgh in 1957. In 1961 he emigrated to the U. S. and became a resident in general surgery at the New England Medical Center in Boston. In the following year, he became a fellow and ultimately an instructor at Temple University Medical Center in Philadelphia, under the tutelage of Harry E. Bacon, one of the giants in the field, textbook author, and editor-in-chief of the journal, *Diseases of the Colon and Rectum*, for many years.

Dr. Khubchandani remained at Temple for three years, certifying in the specialty of colon and rectal surgery in 1963. Following his years at Temple he moved to Allentown, Pennsylvania, where he established one of the country's pre-eminent centers of colon and rectal surgery. It would require more time than I have been allotted for this space if I were to enumerate all of his accomplishments. Dr. Khubchandani is a member of numerous organizations throughout the world. He is a Professor of Surgery at Pennsylvania State University/Hershey Medical Center. He has served on virtually every committee in his hospitals, in the American Society of Colon and Rectal Surgeons, and has served as a reviewer for more than a dozen journals. He has been active in a host of community organizations in Allentown and in India. He has been honored as an Honorary Fellow of the Brazilian, Chilean, Venezuelan, Egyptian, Spanish, Cuban, and Italian Societies of Coloproctology, among many other named professorships, awards, and recognitions. An endowed chair of Colon and Rectal Surgery has been established in his name at Penn State University/Hershey Medical School, at the Lehigh Valley Hospital. He has been the driving force for the establishment and the remarkable growth and recognition of the International Society of University Colon and Rectal Surgeons, wherein he serves as Director General.

In this second edition, the authors have strived to address the needs of the surgeon in training, general surgeons, and colon and rectal surgeons. The concept has been to place into context the numerous recent innovations in the management of hemorrhoidal disease. Simply stated there has been a plethora of newer approaches that have been developed in the last decade, modifications and techniques which are often at considerable odds with oldest surgeons' understanding of the classical approach to the management of this condition—that is, excisional surgery and its technical variations remove hemorrhoidal tissue.

The Contributors represent a who's who in the international community of colon and rectal surgeons. Forty-two surgeons are represented in this otherwise modest-sized book. Fully 13 are from American institutions, but the authors are well distributed internationally. Other countries and institutions include Italy, St. Marks Hospital, Harrow, England, Mexico City, Wycombe, The John Radcliffe Infirmary, Oxford, England, Sao Paulo, Brazil, Vienna, Austria, Singapore, Cairo, Egypt, and Stockholm, Sweden. Without doubt there is a conscientious effort to explore the opinions of numerous individuals with diverse interests in the management of this condition.

The monograph begins with the obligatory series of chapters on history, anatomy, physiology, examination, differential diagnosis, etc. There follows a series of chapters on various techniques which represent essentially historical or antiquated operations, such as the Lord Anal Dilatation, an operation that I believe has essentially fallen into disuse if not disrepute. The same made by said for the Parks Hemorrhoidectomy and Cryotherapy. A number of other chapters discuss more conventional operations. These include a discussion on Transanal Hemorrhoidal Dearterialization, and hemorrhoidectomy using the Ligasure^{TM} vessel sealing system.

Marvin L. Corman, M.D.
Stony Brook University, October 16, 2008

Preface

Much has happened in the management of hemorrhoidal disease since the First Edition was published under the able leadership of Dr. Charles Mann. Some procedures have been delegated as "historical" and have become obsolete by virtue of the data collected, particularly in the era of evidence-based medicine. Other innovations have developed with the help of sophisticated technology. The editors have made an attempt to put together a group of internationally renowned experts, each with personal published data to corroborate their expertise.

The paradigm of management of hemorrhoidal disease has shifted over the years. Surgical excision is relegated to very few advanced cases. The majority of hemorrhoidal diseases can be managed in the office with painless, simple care. When surgery is indicated, "day surgery" has become a standard around the world. The ambulatory hemorrhoidectomy is truly ambulatory, with most patients being discharged for recovery at home within hours of performing the procedure.

The chapters are short, concise, and written with precision. Few tables are utilized and only diagrams which add to the text are included.

It is the editors' fervent desire that the book be palatable to surgical trainees, general surgeons, and colon and rectal surgeons. Where necessary, the description is detailed enough to impart knowledge beyond a cursory narrative.

We are grateful to the contributors, who have given of their time and shared their expertise without any monetary contribution.

Indru Khubchandani, MD (Editor)
Nina Paonessa, DO (Editor)
Khawaja Azimuddin, MD (Editor)

Contents

Contributors

Jeffrey Albright, MD
San Diego, CA
USA

Donato F Altomare, MD
Department of Emergency and Organ
    Transplantation
University of Bari
Bari
Italy

Salim Amrani, MD
Department of General Surgery
State University of New York
Stony Brook, New York
USA

Khawaja Azimuddin, MD, FASCRS
Department of Surgery
Houston, TX
USA

H. Randolph Bailey, MD, FACS
Colon and Rectal Clinic
Houston, TX
USA

Philip F. Caushaj, MD
The Western Pennsylvania Hospital
Department of Surgery
Pittsburgh, PA
USA

Elias Chousleb, MD
Division of Colon and Rectal Surgery
Western Pennsylvania Hospital
Pittsburgh, PA
USA

Soni Chousleb, MD
Division of Colon and Rectal Surgery
Western Pennsylvania Hospital
Pittsburgh, PA
USA

Marvin L. Corman, MD
Department of Surgery
Stony Brook University
Stony Brook, NY
USA

Matthew J. Eckert, MD
Resident, General Surgery
Madigan Army Medical Center
Tacoma, WA
USA

Mr S. Ellesmore
Department of Surgery
St Marks Hospital
Harrow, Middlesex
UK

Javier H. Figueroa-Becerra, MD
Department of General Surgery
Hospital "General José Maria Morelos y
    Pavón" ISSSTE
Mexico City, Mexico

Daniel O. Herzig, MD
Assistant Professor of Surgery
Colorectal Cancer Assessment and Risk Eva-
    luation Clinic (CCARE)
Center for Health & Healing
Portland, OR
USA

Indru T. Khubchandani, MD, FACS, FRCS
Professor of Surgery
Penn State University at Hershey
Adjunct Professor of Surgery
Drexel University at Hahnemann,
    Philadelphia
Division of Colon and Rectal Surgery
Allentown, PA
USA

Dr Edmund I. Leff, MD
Department of Surgery
Scottsdale Healthcare
Scottsdale, Arizona
USA

Mr Peter H Lord (Emeritus)
Wycombe General Hospital
Wycombe
England

Paul A. Lucha Jr., DO, FACOS
Department of General Surgery
Division of Colon and Rectal Surgery
Portsmouth, VA
USA

Martin A. Luchtefeld, MD
Ferguson Clinic - MMPC
Spectrum Health Hospital System
Grand Rapids, MI
USA

Yasuko Maeda, MRCS
Department of Surgery
St Mark's Hospital
Harrow, Middlesex
UK

Charles V Mann (Emeritus)
Section of Coloproctology of the Royal
  Society of Medicine
London
UK

Ramaz Metreveli, MD, PhD, FACS
Department of Surgery
Christiana Care Health System
Wilmington, DE
USA

Pier Paolo Dal Monte, MD
Department of Surgery
Villalba Hospital
Pianoro, Bo
Italy

Abel Morales-Diaz, MD
Unit of Coloproctology
Hospital Angeles Mocel
México City, Mexico

Professor Neil James Mortensen, MD, FRCS
Department of Colorectal Surgery
John Radcliffe Hospital
Oxford
UK

Nina J. Paonessa, DO, FACOS
Clinical Assistant Professor of Surgery
Penn State University at Hershey
Division of Colon and Rectal Surgery
Allentown, PA
USA

Robin K S Phillips, MS, FRCS
Department of Surgery
St Mark's Hospital
Harrow, Middlesex
UK

John J. O'Connor, MD
Department of Surgery
Suburban Hospital
Bethesda, Maryland
USA

José Alfredo dos Reis Junior, MASCRS, FISUCRS, FSBCP
Department of Coloproctology
Clinica Reis Neto
Campinas, Sao Paulo
Brazil

Jose Alfredo dos Reis Neto, FASCRS, FISUCRS, FACF, FRSM, FSBCP, ECBC
Department of Coloproctology
Clinica Reis Neto
Catholic University Pu de Campinas
Campinas, Sao Paulo
Brazil

Irfan Rizvi, MD
Ferguson Clinic – MMPC
Spectrum Health Hospital System
Grand Rapids, MI
USA

Sebastian Roka, MD
Department of General Surgery
General Hospital Vienna
Vienna
Austria

Fidel Ruiz-Healy, MD
Department of Coloproctology
Centro Hospitalario Sanatorio Durango
Mexico City, D.F.
Mexico

Andreas Salat, MD
Department of Surgery, Division of General
  Surgery
Medical University Vienna
Vienna
Austria

Francis Seow-Choen, MBBS, FRCSEd, FAMS
Seow-Choen Colorectal Centre
Mt Elizabeth Hospital
Singapore

Ahmed Shafik[†], MD, PhD
Department of Surgery and Experimental Research,
Cairo University
Cairo
Egypt

Mattias Soop, MD, PhD
Ersta Hospital
Karolinska Institute
Stockholm
Sweden

Scott R. Steele, MD, FACS
Department of Surgery
Madigan Army Medical Center
Fort Lewis, WA

Kok-Yang Tan, MBBS, MMed, FRCS, FAMS
Department of General Surgery
Alexandra Hospital
Singapore

Bela Teleky, MD
Department of Surgery
Medical University Vienna
Vienna
Austria

Michael Warner, MB ChB, FRACS
Department of Colorectal Surgery
John Radcliffe Hospital
Oxford
UK

Mr Alastair C. J. Windsor
The London Clinic
London
UK

Bruce G. Wolff, MD, FACS, FACRS
Department of Colon and Rectal Surgery
Mayo Clinic College of Medicine
Rochester MN
USA

1 Surgical History of Haemorrhoids

S. Ellesmore and A.C.J. Windsor

For as long as man has been blessed with an anus, it is fair to assume that he has also been doubly blessed with haemorrhoids. The word "haemorrhoid" is derived from the Greek *haema* (blood) and *rhoos* (flowing), and it was probably Hippocrates (460 BC) who was the first to apply the name to the flow of blood from the veins of the anus. The term "piles" is derived from the Latin *pila* (a ball) and was widely used by the public at the time of John of Arderne (born AD 1307), and in his treatise of 1370 he remarks that the "common people call them piles, the aristocracy call them haemorrhoids, the French call them figs (*figer*, to clot), what does it matter so long as you can cure them". If only it was that simple.

The Egyptians

Although Egyptian writings left no specific reference to haemorrhoids, there are several descriptions which are unlikely to be any other condition. The *Edwin Smith Papyrus* (1700 BC) (Breasted, 1930) and the Ebers Papyrus (1500 BC) (Ebbel, 1937) both contain references to anal pathology and the *Edwin Smith Papyrus* reports, "if thou inspecteth a man in his anus, whether standing or sitting, suffering very greatly with seizures in both his legs. Thou shouldst give a recipe, an ointment of great protection; Acacia leaves, ground, titurated and cooked together. Smear a strip of fine linen therewith and place in the anus, that he may recover immediately".

The Greeks

The Hippocratic Treatises (460 BC) (Adams, 1849) provide some of the earliest details of both clinical description and surgical treatment of haemorrhoids and in the following reference, Hippocrates is seen to favour an operation to simply ligate the pile: "And haemorrhoids in like manner you may treat by transfixing them with a needle and tying them with very thick and woollen thread; for thus the cure will be the more certain. When you have secured them, use a septic application, and do not foment until they drop off, and always leave one behind; and when the patient recovers let him be put on a course of Hellebore." Further writings "On Haemorrhoids" (Adams, 1849) attributed to Hippocrates deal with haemorrhoidal excision and give mention to an expanding speculum akin to one found in the ruins of Pompeii, and remarkable similar to the Eisenhammer retractor of today. There also appears an interesting description of the aetiology of haemorrhoids: "The disease of the haemorrhoids is formed in this way: if bile or phlegm be determined to the veins of the rectum, it heats the

I. Khubchandani et al. (eds.), *Surgical Treatment of Hemorrhoids*, DOI 10.1007/978-1-84800-314-9_1,

blood in the veins; and being gorged the inside of the gut swells outwardly, and the heads of the veins are raised up, and being at the same time bruised by the faeces passing out, and injured by the blood collected in them, they squirt out blood, most frequently along with the faeces". It is good to see that our understanding of the aetiology of haemorrhoids has improved, though some would question by how much.

The Romans

A Roman contribution to the history of the haemorrhoid is provided by Celsus (25 BC–AD 14). In *De Medicina* (Celsus & Cornelius, 1938), he gives a description of the surgery, mentioning both the ligature and ligature-excision technique, and also mentions the postoperative complication of urinary retention. Galen (AD 131–201) also gives a good clinical description of haemorrhoidal disease, and advocates ligation of haemorrhoids for two hours when surgery is indicated. The intermittent occlusion of the vascular pedicle was also used in the nineteenth century to reduce pain and to avoid spreading gangrene.

The Far East

The only reference of note from Indian medical history is in *The Susruta Samhita* (Bhishnagratna, 1907), the ancient Sanskrit text of Hindu medicine. Opinions are divided as to its date, from fourth century BC to fifth century AD. The work is the Aryan equivalent of the Hippocratic Treatise, but is more surgically advanced. Of note are its emphasis on wound cleanliness and advanced surgical technique.

Following the collapse of the Roman and Greek civilisations, medical knowledge was nurtured by the Arab Empire; Rhazes (AD 860–932), Ali Abbas (AD c.994) and Avicenna (AD 980–1036) (Adams, 1844) all describe the classical operations

for piles. However, the Arab scholars held the baton of medical knowledge for only a short time before returning it to Europe.

The Master Surgeons

At this time Europe was to see one of its finest periods of surgical advancement in the hands of the Master Surgeons. Theodoric (AD 1205–1296) trained at the University of Salerno, discarded Galenical doctrine and advocated healing by primary intention. Lanfrank (died AD 1315) of Milan migrated to Paris in 1295 and became the first great teacher of French surgery. Henri de Mondeville, Guy de Chauliac and John of Arderne (one of the most celebrated early colorectal surgeons), all educated at Montpelier, greatly advanced surgery in a pre-Renaissance revival. Interestingly, master surgeons wrote little during this period, and even less about the management of haemorrhoids. Henri de Mondeville (1260–1320) mentioned haemorrhoids only to warn against operating on them. Unfortunately, the era of the Master Surgeon came to an end with the practise of surgery by the barber and not the scholar; a situation that would remain until the middle of the eighteenth century.

The Barber Surgeons

The era of the barber surgeon lasted for nearly 350 years, and what writings there were from true surgeons were sadly very traditional. The notable surgeons of the time, Ambrose Pare (1510–1590), Master Peter Lowe (1612), Dr Read (1650) and Richard Wiseman (1622–1676), added little to the medical knowledge of haemorrhoids. In polite society at this time, the condition was known as "le mal de St Phiacre", an attempt to confer respectability by the possession of a patron saint; however, there seems to be some doubt about the appropriateness of the chosen patron who was the patron saint of gardeners!

The Renaissance

The eighteenth century saw the end of the barber surgeon and a return of science to medicine. Lorenz Heister (1739) published a work on *Chirurgie*, one of the first textbooks to contain detailed illustrations. He states on haemorrhoids, "but the moderns judging the methods of the ancients too cruel, and often pernicious, generally leave the case to nature, except when the discharge is profuse...". He described ligature with excision, "he is then to tie up the bleeding tunercles with a needle and thread, cutting off those parts which are distended beyond the ligature, taking care at the same time to leave a few of the smallest veins open as before observed".

In the same period, Morgagni (1749) (Morgagni, 1769) published his theory on the aetiology of haemorrhoids, differing from the Hippocratic dogma held by the ancient and mediaeval writers. Morgagni stated, "without doubt, it was not very easy for the blood to pass through a liver of that kind [cirrhotic]. But why, then, you will say, did it not stagnate equally in the other veins which go to the trunk of the vena portarum? And for this very reason it was that I said you would immediately understand it, or at least in part. Add therefore, to omit other things, the very great length, which is peculiar to this one vein [the superior haemorrhoidal] among the others, so that it is much more difficult for the blood to be carried upwards, from this vein, than from the others, especially as the situation of the human body requires it, which without doubt is one of the reasons why other animals are not subject to piles. And if you ask why, in those bodies in which there is any impediment to the quick motion of the blood upwards, the veins of the legs in particular are dilated into varices, you will find the same thing to be the cause of them chiefly which we assign for the piles."

The Nineteenth Century

At the end of the eighteenth century and the beginning of the nineteenth century, men such as Per-civall Pott, William Cheselden and John Hunter created an environment in which writing was encouraged, although interestingly none of these men wrote about haemorrhoids themselves. There was great debate about the relative values of ligation and of excision of haemorrhoids, neither without mortality, and ligation with the added morbidity of intense pain. It would appear that the surgeons of the time had not differentiated between the sensitive anal skin and the insensitive rectal mucosa.

Jean Louis Petit, who wrote a three-volume book on surgery in 1774 (Petit, 1774), rejected excision due to potentially fatal haemorrhage and anal stenosis, and ligation due to pain and gangrene. He noted that the skin of the anus was sensitive and therefore recommended excision ligation, and in 1835, Brodie (Brodie, 1836), in writing about the problems of ligation alone, stated: "The application of the ligature to internal piles in general causes but little pain, and only a slight degree of inflammation follows, for the mucous membrane has nothing like the sensibility of the skin, and does not resent an injury in like manner". In a *Dictionary of Practical Surgery*, Samuel Cooper (1809) both quoted and supported Petit's favour of excision/ligation and, although the technique was not universally accepted, one has to remember that this was before the advent of general anaesthesia and this technique took longer to perform than both excision and ligation alone. Sir Astley Cooper (1836) supported ligation, following the death of three of his patients on whom he had performed an excision – two from bleeding, one from peritonitis – and Copeland described many complications from the excision/ligation technique, including pain, retention of urine, stricture and tetanus. He recommended rectal bouginage, popular with the French schools, thought to treat the increased anal tone which was the cause of haemorrhoids.

The founder of St Marks Hospital, Frederick Salmon, in his short book of rectal surgery (1828), advised bouginage. But we learn later from Allingham (1888) that Salmon modified the excision/ligation operation, incising the perianal skin, dissecting between the haemorrhoidal plexus and the anal musculature as high as the rectal mucosa, then ligating the pedicle.

Little has been added to the operation of haemorrhoidectomy since then, the exception being Whitehead's (1882) operation which involved removing the pile-bearing area of the anal canal and restoring mucosal continuity by the suturing of rectal mucosa to anal skin. It was not adopted in the UK due to the side-effects of stricture, incontinence due to loss of sensation, and soiling due to the presence of rectal mucosa in the anal canal, although it enjoyed greater popularity in America.

The Twentieth Century

The success and safety of Salmon's operation sounded the death knell of the ligation alone technique. Many surgeons have modified this operation since, but none has altered the technique to any great extent. Those worthy of mention are Smith (1876), Alfred Cooper (1887), Quain (1854), Bryant (1861), Goodsall (Goodsall & Miles, 1900), Wallis (1907), Cripps (1884), Ball (1908), Miles (1919), Lockhart-Mummery (1923), Gabriel (1948), Devine (Devine & Devine, 1948), and, of course, the modification described by Milligan, Morgan, et al. (Milligan et al., 1937).

The end of the twentieth century saw two further developments; the diathermy haemorrhoidectomy, as described by Alexander-Williams (Sharif et al., 1991), and the stapled haemorrhoidectomy, using either a linear or a circular stapling device (Longo, 1998). All the various techniques are presently practised and supported by different surgeons, and, as yet, no one technique has proved superior to the others or been universally adopted. The debate as to the aetiology of haemorrhoids continues, with currently accepted theories including varicosity of the anal submucosal veins, vascular hyperplasia and downward displacement of the anal canal lining. It seems logical that a better understanding of aetiology may allow a more appropriate and effective surgical approach.

Conservative Management

The history of haemorrhoids would not be complete without mention of the more conservative treatments we all practise on a daily basis. In 1657, Riverius (Riviere, 1657) was supposed to have used the topical application of nitric acid, a technique reintroduced by Houston (1843). In 1860, quacks were injecting phenol solution into piles, a technique later adopted by the medical profession, after Andrews (1879) thought it to be too dangerous to be used by the quacks.

Cauterisation was revised by Cusack, using a special clamp. This clamp was later modified by Smith, Allingham and von Langenbeck, among others.

Banding was introduced by Barron (1963), and, in many outpatient departments, has found favour over injection.

That the haemorrhoid should be featured in the medical literature of the past four thousand years, that patients in the past were prepared to risk death as a complication of surgery, and that present treatments are still far from perfect, implies that there is more to the humble pile than one first imagines.

The authors would like to acknowledge the late Sir Alan Parks, whose seminal article on the surgical history of haemorrhoids has formed the core research material for this chapter (Parks, 1955).

References and Further Reading

Adams F (1844–1847) The seven books of Paulus Aegineta, Book 6, Sec 79, London, 2, p 403

Adams F (1849) The Genuine Works of Hippocrates, London, 1, pp 333, 825

Allingham W (1888) Diagnosis and Treatment of Disease of the Rectum, Fifth edition, London. Revised by Allingham HW, p 143

Andrews E (1879) Med Rec N Y 15:451

Ball CB (1908) The Rectum, its Diseases and Developmental Defects, London, p 210

Barron J (1963) Office ligation for internal haemorrhoids. Am J Surg 105:563–70

Bhishnagratna KKL (1907) An English Translation of the Susruta Samhita, Calcutta, 2, p 316

Breasted JH (1930) The Edwin Smith Surgical Papyrus, Chicago, 1, p 507

Brodie B (1836) Thirty-six lectures on disease of the rectum. Lond Med Gaz 18:182

Bryant T (1861) Guy's Hosp Rep, 3 s 7:91

Celsus AC (trans 1938) De Medicina, Book 7, Ch 30, Para 3, Spencer WG (trans), London, 3, p 465

Cooper AP (1836) The Principles and Practice of Surgery, London, p 426

Cooper S (1809) A Dictionary of Practical Surgery, London, p 367

Cooper, A (1887) A Practical Treatise on the Diseases of the Rectum, London

Cripps H (1884) On Diseases of the Rectum and Anus, London, p 52

Devine HB, Devine J (1948) The Surgery of the Colon and Rectum, Bristol, p 323

Ebbel B (1937) The Papyrus Ebers, Stockholm, pp 43–4

Gabriel WB (1948) The Principles and Practice of Rectal Surgery, Fourth Edition, London

Galen Galeni Opera ex Octava luntarum. Editone Venetiis apud luntas, MDCIX

Goodsall DH, Miles WE (1900) Diseases of the Anus and Rectum, London

Heister L (1739) A General System of Surgery. Book 5, p 249

Houston J (1843) Dublin J Med Sci 23:95

Lockhart-Mummery JP (1923) Diseases of the Rectum and Colon, London

Longo A (1998) Mundozzi Editore, p 777

Miles WE (1919) Surg Gynecol Obstet 29:497

Milligan ETC, Morgan CN, Jones LE, Officer R (1937) Lancet 2:1119

Morgagni JB (trans 1769) Seats and Causes of Disease, Letter 32, Article 10, Alexander B (trans), London, 2, p 105

Parks AG (1955) De Haemorrhois, a study in surgical history. Guy's Hosp Rep 104:135–56

Petit JL (1774) Traite de Maladies Chirurgicales et des Operations, Paris, 2, p 137

Quain R (1854) The Diseases of the Rectum, London

Riviere L (1657) Praxis Medica cum Theoria Lugduni, Ninth Edition, Book 10, Ch 10, p 184

Salmon F (1828) A Practical Essay on Strictures of the Rectum, Third edition, London, p 205

Sharif HI, Ling Lee, Alexander-Williams (1991) Int J Colorect Dis 6:217–19

Smith H (1876) The Surgery of the Rectum, Fourth Edition, London

Wallis FC (1907) Surgery of the Rectum, London, p 47

Whitehead W (1882) Br Med J 1:148

2 Surgical Anatomy of Hemorrhoids

Ahmed Shafik[†]

Introduction

It is surprising that, in this era of advanced medical achievements, the etiology of one of the commonest human afflictions is not exactly known. Many theories have been advanced regarding the pathogenesis of hemorrhoids, but none is entirely satisfactory. The result of studies on the surgical anatomy of the anal canal is presented with the object of obtaining a clearer understanding of its function in the light of its anatomic structure. A knowledge of such a structural-functional relationship seems necessary for understanding anal pathologies, including hemorrhoids.

Surgical Anatomy

In a previous study, two hemorrhoidal venous plexuses could be identified: submucosal plexus and adventitial plexus. They are connected by communicating veins.

1. **Submucosal plexus:** The veins in the rectal submucosa were arranged in transverse rings along the whole of the rectum including its neck (Figs. 2.1 and 2.2). However, this configuration faded in the pectinate area to appear as a radiological blush (Fig. 2.1); the plexus in this area seemed to be interrupted by the attachment of the rectal neck (anal canal) cutaneous lining to the medial septum of the central tendon. Small side branches came out of the venous rings and penetrated the rectal muscle coat into the adventitia where they collected into multiple oblique veins to form the adventitial plexus. The submucosal plexus consisted of the three hemorrhoidal veins: superior, middle, and inferior; the sites of intercommunication of these veins could not be identified in the submucosa.

2. **Adventitial plexus:** This comprises oblique and vertically lying veins which intercommunicated, forming a plexus in the adventitia of the rectum and its neck (Figs. 2.3 and 2.4). The veins were larger than those of the submucosal plexus. The plexus was drained by the three hemorrhoidal veins; the sites of their communication could be identified. It was formed in the upper half of the rectum by branches of the superior hemorrhoidal vein, and in the lower half by both the superior and middle hemorrhoidal veins; whereas in the rectal neck it was formed by all three of the hemorrhoidal veins. Around the middle of the rectal neck, 3–6 oblique and sizeable "collecting veins" could be identified in the rectal adventitia. They collected into two veins which ascended on the sides to the back of the rectum and united to form the superior hemorrhoidal vein (Figs. 2.4 and 2.5).

3. **Communicating veins:** Two types of communicating veins were recognized: interhemorrhoidal and hemorrhoidogenital.

I. Khubchandani et al. (eds.), *Surgical Treatment of Hemorrhoids*, DOI 10.1007/978-1-84800-314-9_2,
© Springer-Verlag London Limited 2009

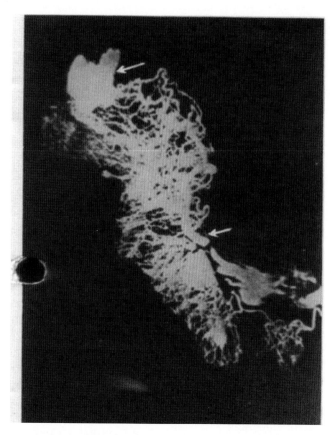

Figure 2.1. Cadaveric specimen showing the barium sulphate solution injected into the inferior mesenteric vein. It demonstrates that the rectal submucosal plexus extends alomg the whole of the rectum including its neck and is arranged in transverse venous rings. The upper arrow points to the superior hemorrhoidal vein.

(a) **Interhemorrhoidal veins:** The three hemorrhoidal veins intercommunicated in the submucosa at the capillary level, and in the adventitia of the rectum and its neck. Yet the exact communication site between the superior and middle hemorrhoidal veins in the submucosa could not be recognized, because the submucosal plexus extended uniformly down to the pectinate line (Fig. 2.1). The blush area below this line seemed to point to the inferior hemorrhoidal plexus (Fig. 2.4). However, in the rectal adventitia the communication sites were easily identified at the rectal neck between the three veins, and around the lower third of the rectum between the superior and middle hemorrhoidal veins.

(b) **Hemorrhoidogenital veins:** This is the name we gave to small veins which connected the adventitial hemorrhoidal with the prostatic or vaginal plexus. They varied in number from one to three veins on either side of the upper rectal neck. They lay in the rectal neck adventitia, and passed forward to reach the prostatic base and join the prostatic venous plexus (Figs. 2.2–2.5). In females, the veins proceeded to the side wall of the upper half of the vagina and joined the vaginal plexus. When the inferior mesenteric vein was injected with barium sulphate, the bladder wall in males (Figs. 2.2–2.4) and the vagina, uterus, and bladder in females were opacified through the hemorrhoidogenital

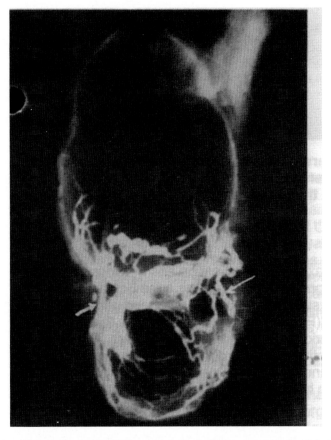

Figure 2.2. Transverse section of the rectum and urinary bladder after injecting the inferior mesenteric vein with barium sulphate and after being inflated with air and frozen. It shows the submucosal rectal plexus arranged in transverse rings. It also shows the hemorrhoidogenital veins (arrow). Observe that the bladder wall is opacified, the dye passing to it through the hemorrhoidogenital veins.

veins. The hemorrhoidogenital veins seemed to be valved, because they were unidirectional. They directed the blue plastic (Astralon) and the barium sulphate suspension from the hemorrhoidal to the prostatic plexus, but not in the reverse direction. Thus, when either of them was injected into the deep dorsal vein of the penis to the prostatic plexus, they could not be recovered in the hemorrhoidal plexus of any patient.

Collecting hemorrhoidal veins: Contrary to views of investigators [1, 2] that the "collecting hemorrhoidal veins" lie in the columns of Morgagni, our study demonstrated that they exist in the rectal adventitia. The columns are only plicate mucosal folds that result from both the fusion of the wide hindgut with the narrow proctodeum and the tonic action of the rectal neck sphincters. Two sites of porto-systemic communication could be identified in the rectum: interhemorrhoidal and hemorrhoidogenital. The first one occurs between the three hemorrhoidal veins, both submucosally and adventitially. The communication site was identified in the adventitia but not in the submucosa. The portal blood is shunted through this communication to the internal iliac vein. The second communication is through the hemorrhoidogenital veins which connect the hemorrhoidal plexus with the prostatic or vaginal one. It seems that this

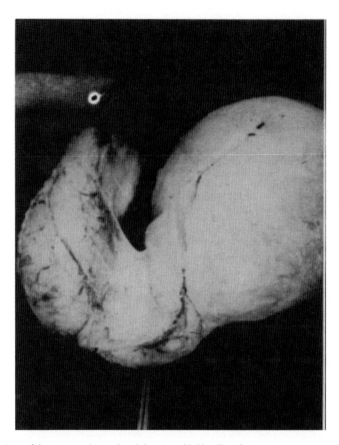

Figure 2.3. Cadaveric specimen of the rectum and its neck and the urinary bladder. The inferior mesenteric vein was injected with blue plastic (Astralon). The artery forceps points to the urethra. The specimen shows the adventitial hemorrhoidal plexus as well as the hemorrhoidogenital veins.

portosystemic connection is sizeable, because the urinary bladder, vagina, and uterus were opacified each time the inferior mesenteric vein was injected with barium sulphate (Figs. 2.2, 2.4, 2.5). In contrast to investigators [1, 2] who mentioned that the hemorrhoidal plexus is located in the lower rectum and anal canal and is only submucosal, the present study demonstrates that not only does it extend along the whole rectum and its neck but it is both submucosal and adventitial.

Being extensive, the plexus can absorb excess venous congestion along its entire length before it becomes varicose; furthermore, the varicosity would involve the whole venous plexus and not only its lower submucosal part. It simulates in this respect the diffuse congestion and varicosity of the pampiniform plexus in varicocele. This fact, and in addition the fact that the portal hemorrhoidal blood can work its way to the systemic circulation through two portosystemic shunts (interhemorrhoidal and hemorrhoidogenital), together tend to negate the theory of venous congestion in the lower part of the hemorrhoidal plexus as the primary event in hemorrhoidogenesis.

Our findings support the conclusion that hemorrhoids are a mucosal prolapse resulting primarily from the constricting effect of the anorectal band on the rectal neck [3]. They explain the rarity of hemorrhoids in portal hypertension; it has been found that the incidence of hemorrhoids in bilharzial liver cirrhosis patients does not differ from that in our normal population [1]. It also explains the

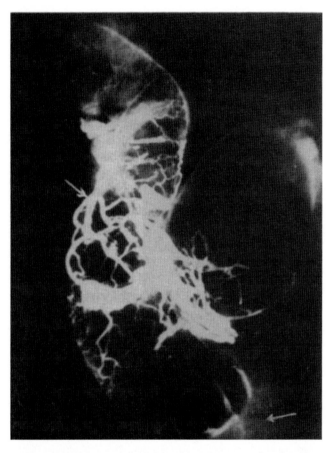

Figure 2.4. Barium sulphate injected into the inferior mesenteric vein. The oblique large veins are those of the adventitial plexus, whereas the upper small transverse veins belong to the submucosal plexus. The pectinate area shows the radiological blush (lower arrow). The bladder wall is opacified through the hemorrhoidogenital veins. The upper arrow points to the superior hemorrhoidal vein.

rarity of rectal bleeding in these patients, compared with esophageal bleeding.

Portosystemic circulation in the rectum: Under normal physiologic conditions, the submucosal hemorrhoidal plexus drains into the adventitial one, and the latter into the three hemorrhoidal veins. Because of the submucosal and adventitial intercommunication of the three veins in the rectal neck, and the presence of the hemorrhoidogenital veins, portal blood may drain into the systemic circulation, particularly when the rectum contracts at defecation. This was proven in a recent study [4] in which a contrast medium was injected into the rectal neck submucosa of normal living subjects; the dye showed in the vesicoprostatic and vesicovaginal plexus. Systemic blood, however, cannot drain into portal blood, as was verified in the present study. When either barium sulphate or blue plastic was injected into the deep dorsal vein of the penis, it could not be recovered in the hemorrhoidal plexus. This is probably due to the presence of valves in the middle and inferior hemorrhoidal veins, which direct the blood to the systemic circulation, and not vice versa. Unlike elsewhere, portal blood shunted from the rectum and left colon to the systemic circulation seems to be harmless from the metabolic viewpoint, because this blood carries no nutritives.

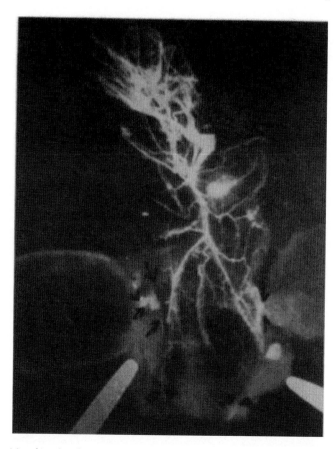

Figure 2.5. Barium sulphate injected into the inferior mesenteric vein. The rectum and urinary bladder were inflated, frozen, and bisected. The artery forceps points to the urethra. The specimen shows the "collecting veins." The upper arrows point to the hemorrhoidogenital veins, through which the bladder wall is opacified. The lower arrows point to the inferior hemorrhoidal plexus.

Arterial pattern of the anorectum: A study of the arterial pattern of the anorectum [6] has shown that the superior rectal artery (SRA) and vein were enclosed in a fibrous sheath which was connected to the posterior rectal surface by an anterior mesorectum containing the "transverse rectal branches," and to the sacrum by an avascular posterior mesorectum (Fig. 2.6). Small lymph nodes were scattered alongside the anterior mesorectum. The SRA gave rise to four branches: transverse rectal, descending rectal, rectosigmoid, and terminal (Figs. 2.6, 2.7). The transverse rectal arteries arose from the SRA in 24 specimens and from the descending rectal artery in eight. They were distributed to the upper half of the rectum. The rectosigmoid artery was distributed to the descending limb of the sigmoid colon and rectosigmoid junction. We found two terminal branches in 21/32 cadavers and three in 11/32. They communicated in the lower half of the rectum. The inferior rectal arteries were present in all the dissected cadavers, while the middle rectal arteries could be identified in only 50% of the cadavers. Two arterial patterns were recognized: annular in the upper rectal half provided by the transverse rectal arteries, and plexiform in the lower half supplied by the SRA terminal branches.

The above anatomical facts lend credence to the theory of hemorrhoidal etiology being arteriovenous communications (corpora cavernosa).

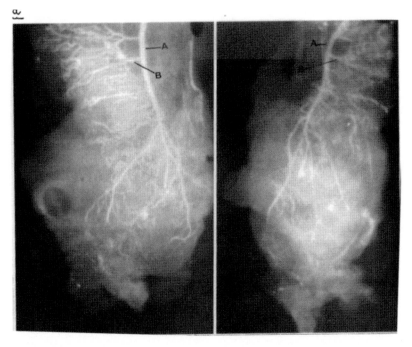

Figure 2.6. Arteriogram showing the SRA (A) giving rise to the transverse rectal branches. (B) The terminal branches of the transverse rectal arteries do not anastomose anteriorly, and this results in the formation of a "bloodless line." The SRA terminates at the mid-rectum, giving rise to three branches. (a) Lateral view. (b) Anteroposterior view.

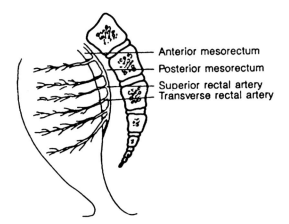

— Anterior mesorectum
— Posterior mesorectum
— Superior rectal artery
— Transverse rectal artery

Figure 2.7. Diagrammatic illustration of the SRA giving rise to the transverse rectal arteries and two terminal branches.

References

1. Goligher JC. Surgery of the anus, rectum and colon. Bailliere Tindall, London, 1980.
2. Goldberg SM, Gordon PH, Nivatvongs S. Essentials of anorectal surgery. Lippincott Co., Philadelphia & Toronto, 1980.
3. Shafik A. The pathogenesis of haemorrhoids and their treatment by anorectal bandotomy. J Clin Gastroenterol 1984;6:129–37.
4. Shafik A. Anal cystography: new technique of cystography. Preliminary report. Urology 1984;23:313–16.
5. Shafik A. Urethral discharge, constipation and haemorrhoids. New syndrome with report of 7 cases. Urology 1981;18:155–60.
6. Shafik A, Moustafa H. Study of the arterial pattern of the rectum and its clinical application. Acta Anat 1996;157:80–86.

3 Pathophysiology of Hemorrhoidal Disease

Paul A. Lucha

Background

The prevalence of hemorrhoidal disease is difficult to determine. Some estimate that up to 90% of patients may complain of hemorrhoidal symptoms at least once in their lifetime [1]. The incidence of hemorrhoids increases with age, with males affected twice as often as females. Age predisposes to a laxity of Treitz's ligaments, with an average onset after age 30. There are hereditary predispositions; however, occupational predisposition has not been demonstrated. Low residue diets seen typically in industrialized countries have been described as contributing to symptomatic hemorrhoids, presumably by causing smaller hard stools. This is clearly not the only etiology however, as those patients with diarrhea may also develop symptomatic hemorrhoids. Diets high in fiber may reduce the risk of hemorrhoid congestion. Although increased intra-abdominal pressure such as that seen in chronic pulmonary disease, prostatism, and pelvic tumors has been postulated to contribute to symptomatic hemorrhoids, the actual incidence is no greater in these patients than is found in the general population.

Data from the National Center for Health Statistics estimate that 10 million people in the United States have had symptomatic hemorrhoids; however, this may actually underestimate the problem, because the majority of patients may not seek professional care, preferring self-medication instead. Those who eventually seek medical care complaining of hemorrhoids often have another reason for their complaint. In one recent audit, only 20% of patients initially believed to have symptomatic hemorrhoids when presenting to their physician actually had hemorrhoids as the etiology of their complaints [2, 3, 4]. The most common presenting symptom is bleeding. It usually happens toward the end of defecation and is often bright red and painless. Prolapse and thrombosis may also occur. The patient may also complain of swelling and itching, but pain may also be present if there is thrombosis involving the external hemorrhoids [1, 5].

Pathophysiology and Anatomy

The anal canal is the terminal portion of the gastrointestinal tract. It begins approximately 2 cm proximal to the dentate line and extends to the anal verge. Anatomists and surgeons differ on the "definition" of the anal canal. The anatomic anal canal starts at the dentate line and extends to the anal verge, whereas the surgical anal canal includes the anatomic anal canal and the tissue 2 cm proximal to the dentate line (see Fig. 3.1). The lining of the surgical anal canal transitions from columnar mucosa above the dentate line to squamous epithelium containing hair follicles and sweat glands at the anal verge. The transitional

I. Khubchandani et al. (eds.), *Surgical Treatment of Hemorrhoids*, DOI 10.1007/978-1-84800-314-9_3,
© Springer-Verlag London Limited 2009

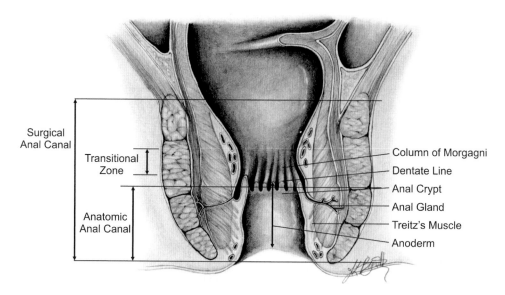

Figure 3.1. Surgical anal canal

zone, 0.5–1 cm above the dentate line, contains an abundance of nerve endings and is responsible for fine sensory discrimination [1, 6].

Hemorrhoids are cushions of vascular tissue arising above the dentate line (insensate) and extending to the anal verge (sensate). Microscopically, hemorrhoids are sinusoids (vascular structures without muscular walls) with a blood supply arising from the middle and inferior rectal arteries. Bleeding from hemorrhoids is arterial, arising from the presinusoidal arterial plexus, as evidenced by the bright red color, and having an arterial pH. The hemorrhoids arise in three main positions: right posterior, right anterior, and left lateral, which is coincident with the terminal branches of the hemorrhoidal vessels. Normal engorgement of these cushions contributes to the maintenance of continence.

It has been suggested that chronic straining secondary to constipation or occasionally diarrhea may result in pathologic hemorrhoids. Eventually, with repeated straining, the hemorrhoids may lose their attachment (Treitz's ligaments) to the underlying rectal wall, leading to the prolapse of the tissue into the anal canal. The engorged tissue becomes more friable, which may contribute to bleeding. These tissues communicate with the superficial

subcutaneous venules at the anal verge, which may result in external hemorrhoidal dilation [6, 7, 8]. Internal hemorrhoids are classified by history and not by physical examination, as follows:

- Grade I—bleeding without prolapse.
- Grade II—prolapse with spontaneous reduction.
- Grade III—prolapse with manual reduction.
- Grade IV—incarcerated, irreducible prolapse.

The utility of this system is that it correlates well with management recommendations; i.e., Grade I and II hemorrhoids are often successfully treated by non-operative means, while Grade III and Grade IV hemorrhoids are more likely to require surgery. Investigators have suggested that those patients with symptomatic hemorrhoids have higher anal canal pressures. Anal canal pressures were measured in symptomatic and asymptomatic patients, demonstrating significantly higher pressures in the symptomatic patients. These patients had a fall in their resting pressures following treatment for the hemorrhoids, but still remained higher than asymptomatic controls. The magnitude of the pressure elevation did not correlate with the duration of symptoms or degree of prolapse [9, 10, 11, 12].

Treatment Options

Early disease (Grade I and early Grade II) is often managed with medications designed to cause vaso-constriction and treat inflammation for the engorged friable hemorrhoid. More advanced disease frequently requires operative management which may include sclerotherapy, cryosurgery, infrared coagulation, rubber band ligation, and various modes of surgical excision. These therapies attempt to remove the redundant tissue and create cicatrices to fix the remaining mucosa within the anal canal once again.

References

1. Marti M-C. Hemorrhoids. In: Marti M-C, Givel J-C, eds. Surgery of anorectal diseases. Springer-Verlag 1990:56–75.
2. Rohde H, Christ H. Haemorrhoids are too often assumed and treated. Survey of 548 patients with anal discomfort. Dtsch Med Wochenschr 2004;129:1965–69.
3. Johanson JF, Sonnenberg A. The prevalence of hemorrhoids and chronic constipation. An epidemiologic study. Gastroenterology 1990;98:380–86.
4. Cataldo PA. Hemorrhoids. ASCRS Core Subjects 2005. <http://www.fascrs.org>.
5. Sack J. Pathophysiology of hemorrhoidal disease. Sem Colon Rectal Surg 2003;14:93–99.
6. Trudel J. Anatomy and physiology of the colon, rectum, and anus. ASCRS Core Subjects 2003. <http://www.fascrs.org>.
7. Haas PA, Fox TA, Haas GP. Pathogenesis of hemorrhoids. Dis Colon Rectum 1984;7:442–50.
8. Beck D. Hemorrhoidal disease. In: Beck DE and Wexner SD, eds. Fundamentals of anorectal surgery, 2nd ed. WB Saunders 1998:237–53.
9. Deutsch AA, Moshkovitz M, Nudelman I, Dinari G, Reiss R. Anal pressure measurements in the study of hemorrhoid etiology and their relation to treatment. Dis Colon Rectum 1987;30:855–57.
10. Sun WM, Read NW, Shorthouse AJ. Hypertensive anal cushions as a cause of the high anal canal pressures in patients with haemorrhoids. Br J Surg 1990; 77:458–62.
11. Hiltunen KM, Matikainen M. Anal manometric findings in symptomatic hemorrhoids. Dis Colon Rectum 1985; 28:807–09.
12. Waldron DJ, Kumar D, Hallan RI, Williams NS. Prolonged ambulant assessment of anorectal function in patients with prolapsing hemorrhoids. Dis Colon Rectum 1989; 32:968–74.

4 Diagnosis

Khawaja Azimuddin

The diagnosis of hemorrhoids is simple but often tricky. Perhaps there is no other condition that is as often misdiagnosed as hemorrhoids. Both patients and physicians tend to blame "hemorrhoids" for a multitude of problems in the anorectal area, often with dangerous consequences. I have seen many cases where "hemorrhoids" were blamed for the patient's symptoms and even treated for years, when the actual pathology was either a fissure, fistula, prolapse, anal papilla, or in some cases even a carcinoma.

It should be made clear right at the outset that the diagnosis of "hemorrhoids" should be reached only after confirming the hemorrhoids on visual and anoscopic examination and only after other sources of anorectal symptoms have been excluded. Needless to say, if a proper history is taken and a complete anorectal exam is performed, there should be no difficulty in reaching the correct diagnosis.

As with any other medical condition, diagnosis requires a proper history and a detailed physical examination [1]. A properly taken history and physical exam will not only help make the diagnosis of hemorrhoids but also steer the surgeon towards making the correct treatment choice for a particular patient. In my opinion, the true caliber of a colorectal surgeon can be judged not by his degrees but by the care and expertise he demonstrates in the diagnosis of common anorectal ailments such as hemorrhoids.

History

History taking should not be considered a menial task delegated to the most junior member of the team. Instead, a thorough and systematic approach should be taken. History should be directed not only towards the symptomatology of hemorrhoids and confirming the diagnosis but also towards excluding other more sinister conditions. In addition, a proper history should assist the colorectal surgeon in making the appropriate decisions for the treatment of hemorrhoids.

The surgeon should inquire about the nature, duration, and severity of symptoms and the extent of discomfort the hemorrhoids are causing. It is also important to get a good idea about what the patient's expectations are. Certainly a patient who has an occasional asymptomatic prolapse and is otherwise not incapacitated by the disease may not want a painful recovery from an excisional hemorrhoidectomy.

Most patients with hemorrhoids have symptoms for a long period of time before they seek medical attention. Often the patients have self-diagnosed the problem and have spent months or even years trying to treat themselves with over the counter medications or ointments. Some patients, however, especially those with a nervous predisposition, present early or even after a single episode of bright red rectal bleeding. While taking the history, the proctologist should focus on the following aspects:

I. Khubchandani et al. (eds.), *Surgical Treatment of Hemorrhoids*, DOI 10.1007/978-1-84800-314-9_4,
© Springer-Verlag London Limited 2009

Age: Most patients who develop hemorrhoids are between the ages of 30 and 50. In patients who present at an unusually early age, extra care should be exercised in excluding other diagnostic possibilities such as inflammatory bowel disease, juvenile polyps, polyposis syndromes, etc. On the other hand, in older patients, the diagnosis of carcinoma should always be borne in mind.

Gender: Hemorrhoids occur in both sexes. However, pregnancy and childbirth are the prime causes of hemorrhoids in young females. The hormonal milieu of pregnancy, venous congestion, and increased pelvic pressure in late pregnancy and delivery all contribute to the development of hemorrhoids. Once the pregnancy is over, the hemorrhoids tend to improve over the next few months.

Medical history: Some patients with leukemia or bleeding diathesis will have complications from hemorrhoids. Others may be on anticoagulants, nonsteroidal anti-inflammatory drugs, or Plavix®. These patients will also have a tendency to bleed. If surgery is being contemplated, these drugs will have to be stopped before surgery. Patients who smoke should be counseled to stop before surgery.

Family history: Family history should include questions directed towards excluding familial colorectal neoplastic syndromes. In certain individuals, there may be a genetic predisposition towards development of hemorrhoids. The vein walls or venous valves may be weak. These patients will have a positive family history of hemorrhoid problems.

Bowel habits: (a) Excessive straining will predispose to hemorrhoids. Some individuals habitually strain for a bowel movement. Such constant pressure causes engorgement and stretching of the vascular anal cushions. Ultimately the supporting connective tissue holding the vascular cushions is stretched and broken and the vascular cushions slide downward, presenting as hemorrhoids. (b) Some patients with chronic constipation suffer from hemorrhoid problems. It is not clear if constipation causes hemorrhoids but constipation and straining can certainly aggravate

hemorrhoids. The combination of constipation and "hemorrhoids" should always raise the possibility of a low-lying rectal cancer. (c) On the other hand, patients with chronic diarrhea also develop hemorrhoids. Tenesmus from diarrhea does cause straining, and the constant irritation from loose stools will also damage the delicate hemorrhoidal veins. The combination of diarrhea and hemorrhoids should also raise the possibility of inflammatory bowel disease.

Dietary habits: The surgeon should enquire about the adequate intake of water and fiber in diet. Lack of fiber in diet is perhaps the most common predisposing factor in the development of hemorrhoids. The intake of constipating foods such as cheese and milk should be ascertained. On the other hand, diarrhea may be caused by beer, citrus fruits, lactose intolerance, and caffeine, once again aggravating the symptoms of hemorrhoids. Treatment of hemorrhoids without correcting these simple factors is doomed to fail.

Social history: It is important to enquire about social issues and lifestyle before embarking upon treatment of hemorrhoids. Treatment of hemorrhoids without correcting these factors is destined to failure: (a) Spending hours or reading books on the bathroom commode, while attempting to defecate, is an ominous sign, and any operative treatment in these patients is doomed to fail unless the habit is broken before embarking upon surgery. If the patient continues to strain for defecation after surgery, the hemorrhoids are sure to recur. (b) Some athletes, such as weight lifters and tennis players, exert themselves in extreme bursts of muscular activity which raises the intra-abdominal pressure and can be associated with prolapse of internal hemorrhoids or thrombosis of external hemorrhoids. (c) Hemorrhoids may also become aggravated and irritated in patients who practice anorectal intercourse. In these patients, it is important to exclude other diseases such as abscess, fissure, or ulcers, and to evaluate the immune system before undertaking treatment. (d) Prolonged sitting and lack of activity has also been reported to predispose to hemorrhoids.

Previous treatment: Any previous surgery may impact upon the anatomy and function of the anorectum. Therefore, before offering treatment, the colorectal surgeon must enquire about any previous operations: (a) In a patient who has had a previous internal sphincterotomy or fistulotomy, surgery may result in fecal incontinence by further compromising the sphincter function. In some patients the bulk of the hemorrhoidal cushions may even be aiding in maintaining continence. Once these are removed, incontinence may be unmasked. Such patients may be better off with conservative measures such as fiber supplements or at most rubber bandings. (b) In patients with a properly performed previous hemorrhoidectomy, recurrence is usually limited and isolated. Such patients may be best managed with conservative measures such as banding or ligation. A repeat hemorrhoidectomy should be performed with utmost caution, because it may lead to anal stenosis. (c) In patients with previous sclerotherapy, the mucosa is often adherent to the underlying sphincter, making the operation more difficult.

Symptoms

Principal complaints of hemorrhoids include bleeding on defecation and prolapse of tissue. Secondary symptoms may be associated with hemorrhoids but often arise from other causes which are unrelated. Contrary to popular belief, pain is not a primary symptom and usually occurs as a result of complications of hemorrhoids.

Principal Symptoms

Bleeding on Defecation

Rectal bleeding is the most common symptom of hemorrhoids. Hemorrhoidal bleeding is bright red and painless [2]. If there is pain, another diagnosis such as a fissure should be entertained. It usually occurs at or immediately after defecation. It is not mixed with stools. It is usually small in amount but occasionally patients may experience heavy bleeding.

Blood dripping or squirting into the bowl at the end of defecation is highly suggestive of hemorrhoids. Some patients have large prolapsing and vascular hemorrhoids that remain outside and become traumatized as the patient sits on hard surfaces or rides a car. Such patients will complain of spontaneous bleeding and staining of their underwear in between bowel movements. On the other hand, some large fourth-degree hemorrhoids do not bleed because their exposed mucosa becomes thick and calloused. Bleeding unrelated to defecation should always raise the possibility of another pathology such as a carcinoma.

Prolapse

Prolapse is another common symptom of hemorrhoids. It occurs in larger hemorrhoids. Hemorrhoidal prolapse usually occurs at the time of defecation. It is usually painless and reduces spontaneously after defecation. It is such an important feature that the classification of hemorrhoids depends upon the degrees of prolapse [3]. First-degree hemorrhoids do not prolapse. Second-degree hemorrhoids prolapse during defecation but reduce spontaneously. Third-degree hemorrhoids prolapse and have to be reduced manually. Fourth-degree hemorrhoids are trapped outside the anal canal and cannot be reduced by manual pressure. Alternative but less common causes of prolapse include mucosal prolapse, full-thickness rectal prolapse, anterior wall prolapse and fibro-epithelial and adenomatous polyps. These occur independently of defecation and must be excluded before treatment is offered.

Secondary Symptoms

Mucus Discharge

Mucus is produced by the secretory columnar epithelium above the dentate line. When the prolapse is significant enough to protrude through the anal canal, the columnar mucosa is exposed to the outside environment and becomes irritated, thus secreting mucus. It is important to rule out other causes of mucus such as a mucus-secreting rectal villous adenoma, carcinoma, mucosal prolapse, ectropion from previous hemorrhoidectomy, or proctitis.

Pain

Internal hemorrhoids that do not prolapse should not cause pain. Prolapsed hemorrhoids can cause a dragging sensation until they are reduced. Once the prolapse is reduced the discomfort quickly resolves. A prolapse that fails to reduce either spontaneously or manually will become strangulated or thrombosed and will cause severe pain. Apart from these two examples, pain is usually not a feature of hemorrhoids and should raise the possibility of another disease such as a fissure or abscess.

Pruritis

Mucus discharge can cause maceration and irritation of skin leading to pruritis. Most often however pruritis is secondary to other causes such as infections or dermatological conditions.

Anemia

Anemia rarely arises from hemorrhoids. However, I have seen a case of an unfortunate lady who was chronically anemic from recurrent rectal bleeding and was receiving Procrit® on a monthly basis! Numerous gastroenterologists had performed colonoscopies and confirmed internal hemorrhoids on multiple occasions, but the patient was never referred to a surgeon. Needles to say, she never required another shot of Procrit® after I rubber banded her hemorrhoids! Barring these rare exceptions, anemia in a patient with rectal bleeding should raise suspicion of more ominous causes such as a carcinoma.

Altered Bowel Habits

A change in bowel habits or narrowing stool caliber should never be attributed to hemorrhoids. Any patient with hemorrhoids whose bowel habits are abnormal, especially if they have changed, should be thoroughly investigated for alternative diagnoses such as cancer or proctocolitis.

Fecal Incontinence

Some patients with large prolapsing hemorrhoids may complain of minor fecal incontinence. The large chronically prolapsed hemorrhoids may cause incomplete closure of the anal canal and predispose to the leakage of mucus and feces. However as a general rule, fecal incontinence should never be attributed to hemorrhoids. An important cause of incontinence which is often confused with hemorrhoids is rectal prolapse. The proctologist should have a high index of suspicion when a patient with hemorrhoids complains of incontinence. These patients should be examined on a commode while straining to rule out a rectal prolapse.

Physical Examination

Examination should be performed in a private, well illuminated room. The room need not be fancy, but should be equipped with the essential items required for the examination. These include a suction system, a long plastic suction rod, a good portable or head light, and a washing sink. Ideally a toilet should be within the room. Enemas should be readily available in case distal bowel preparation is required. Lubricant jelly and soft tissue paper to wipe off the lubricant is required in all cases. It is important that instruments are within easy reach of the surgeon. These include scalpel, scissors, needle holders and suture materials. Anoscope and proctoscopes should also be available in the room and discreetly covered in order to avoid patient anxiety. 1% Lidocaine with epinephrine, syringes, and small gauge needles should be readily available in case a procedure needs to be performed.

As with the history, the examination is also divided into separate well-defined parts which are described in the following paragraphs.

General Examination

The examination begins with the general appearance of the patient, vital signs, and body weight. It starts at the moment the patient enters the room and is directed towards answering two questions: (1) Is the patient's general appearance and fitness consistent with the simple diagnosis of hemorrhoids? (2) Are the patient's medical comorbidities, personality, and body habitus a contraindication to standard management? Patients with hemorrhoids are generally young, fit, and healthy. Rarely, patients may have anemia or stigmata of liver failure.

If surgery is being considered, additional examinations or tests may be required. A patient with a history of smoking or pulmonary diseases will require a thorough examination of the respiratory system. Patients with a history of hypertension or heart problems will require a cardiac examination. If abnormalities are encountered during the exam, then a further pulmonary or cardiac workup may be warranted before surgery. In patients who will likely need surgery, preoperative blood work, an EKG, or a chest X-ray may be required, according to anesthesia guidelines.

Abdominal Examination

Abdominal examination must be carried out in all patients who present for hemorrhoids. It is most conveniently performed in the supine position just before turning the patient to the left lateral side for the rectal examination. Like all abdominal examinations, it is carried out in a systematic fashion and encompasses all four quadrants.

Special consideration should be given to the following areas: (a) Abdominal distention; this may be secondary to ascites or bowel obstruction. (b) Dilated abdominal wall veins may indicate portal hypertension or blockage of inferior vena cava. (c) Hepatomegaly; this may be secondary to cirrhosis or hepatic metastasis. (d) Splenomegaly; this may be secondary to portal hypertension. (e) Inguinal adenopathy; enlarged lymph nodes in the groin may be from an anal or low rectal malignancy. (f) Abdominal mass; this may be secondary to a gastrointestinal malignancy. (g) Pelvic mass; this could be secondary to an enlarged uterus from pregnancy, fibroids, or uterine or ovarian malignancy.

Some of the above conditions such as GI cancer or anorectal varices may be confused with hemorrhoids. Others such as a pelvic or abdominal mass may be the cause of hemorrhoids by virtue of their back pressure effect on the pelvic venous system.

Preparation

Before proceeding with the examination, an informed consent must be obtained. Since the visual and digital examination usually leads to proctoscopy, anoscopy, and even treatment of hemorrhoids in many instances, it is essential to inform the patient of the possible intervention. In most cases a verbal consent is all that is necessary. However, because of the medico-legal issues that plague our practices these days, it may not be a bad idea to take a written consent before starting the examination.

A complete anorectal examination is possible if there are no feces in the rectum. In most patients, the amount of feces in an unprepared rectum is sufficiently small to allow a proper examination. If the patient has had a bowel movement that morning, the rectum is usually empty.

It is my preference to perform a digital rectal examination and assess the degree of contamination first. If there are minimal stools in the rectum then I proceed with the examination and proctoscopy. On the other hand, if there are solid stools in the rectum, I use a Fleet enema®. It can be easily given in the office and acts promptly, making it suitable for routine use in the office. Stimulant suppositories such as Dulcolax are a possible alternative but are often slow to work and sometimes do not achieve adequate fecal evacuation.

The use of bowel preparation is not without some disadvantages. It can eliminate significant residues such as blood, mucus, or pus from the rectum, thereby depriving the examiner of some important diagnostic clues. Also, it can cause local irritation and proctitis which sometimes leads to overdiagnosis.

Position

An examination is generally performed in either the left lateral, knees up position or the face down, knee-elbow position (Fig. 4.1). Both positions offer certain advantages and disadvantages and there is no evidence that one is superior to the other. The left lateral position, also known as the Sims position, is probably the simplest and does not require a special couch. The patient lies on his left side with the knees and elbows flexed. The buttocks should be brought as close as possible to (and even hanging over) the edge of the table. The hips and knees should be flexed as much as possible. The right knee and hip should be flexed more and brought over the left knee to improve access to the anus. It is my preferred position for examination. It is comfortable for the patients and least embarrassing. In a frail and disabled patient this may be the only position that can be tolerated.

Another advantage is that a patient who is undergoing abdominal examination in the supine position can be simply turned on his side and the examination may continue without interruption.

In the prone jackknife or knee-elbow position the patient kneels down while bracing himself on his elbows or chest. The knee-elbow position has some advantages as well. Patients can easily and quickly assume this position without much difficulty. It separates the buttocks efficiently and enhances access to and gives excellent visualization of the perianal area. By tilting the upper torso forward, it shifts the gastrointestinal contents down hill, away from the anorectum, thereby improving the visualization of the lower rectum and anus. It also assists in straightening out the rectosigmoid angle, which facilitates the passage of the proctoscope.

However, caution must be exercised when using this position in patients with acute glaucoma, severe debilitation, severe arrhythmia, late pregnancy, and recent abdominal surgery [2]. The position can be uncomfortable when employed on a nonadjustable table. It therefore requires a special table with a soft cushioned ledge on which the patient can kneel with the body tilted forward.

Special couches are available for use in coloproctology offices. They are expensive and require extra time for the patient to be properly positioned and secured. Their great advantage is that once the patient is settled in, they are very comfortable and the patient can tolerate a relatively prolonged examination and/or treatment session. However, for most practical purposes, an inexpensive regular examination table with the patient in left lateral position is as effective as any "Cadillac" version.

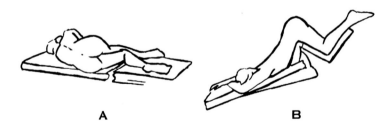

A   **B**

Figure 4.1 (A) Left lateral position (B) Prone jackknife position.

Whatever position is adopted for routine use in the clinic, it should be applied in an accurate and consistently repeatable fashion, which ensures an optimum condition for examination and improves work flow in the office. In particular, it should maximize patient confidence and comfort, allow excellent illumination and visualization of the perineum and anus, permit the examining physician to use instruments and perform procedures, as well as give access to an assistant. In my opinion, the left lateral position fulfills all these criteria.

Because the proctologist may need to spend considerable time conducting the examination and possibly treatment in this position, he or she should be seated comfortably on a stool. The instrument table should be on the right side so that these can be easily picked up while the proctologist remains seated on the examining stool. Alternatively, a nurse who is standing on the right-hand side of the proctologist may pick up the instruments and hand them to the surgeon. An additional nurse, standing on the surgeon's left side, may occasionally be required to hold the buttocks apart or to hold the anoscope if a more involved procedure is being performed.

It is very important to establish a routine and practice it every time so that every one in the office, and even "seasoned" patients, become accustomed to it. This will help to improve the work flow and efficiency in the office. I first sit the patient on the examination table while taking the history. Then the patient is helped to lie in a supine position. The patient is covered with an examining sheet and asked to lift up the hips and pull down the undergarments. An abdominal exam is performed and then I simply ask the patient to turn to the left lateral position. At this stage, a rectal exam is done followed by proctoscopy and anoscopy. The idea is to establish a seamless transition between all phases of the exam and improve flow and efficiency.

Visual Inspection

Once the patient is properly positioned, he or she should be relaxed, comfortable, and able to respond to questions and instructions. It is important to make the patient comfortable by engaging in pleasant and reassuring conversation. He or she should be constantly informed about what is happening and should be continually reassured that they will not experience pain, only discomfort at the worst. If any treatment is planned, he or she should be informed. The proctologist should also be sitting comfortably on an examining stool during the exam and must not rush through the stages of the examination. If the patient's buttocks are bulky, they may obscure visualization. In this case, adhesive tape or an assistant's hands should be employed to retract the overlying folds. Good lighting is essential for the examination and should be focused on the perianal area.

Because visual inspection usually proceeds seamlessly to anoscopy, proctoscopy, and often treatment as well, it is helpful if the instruments are within easy reach and located on the right side on a table that is set at the same height as the sitting proctologist.

Even when the diagnosis of hemorrhoids is almost certain, visual examination starts with the perianal skin and perineum. Inspection is carried out with the patient relaxed but then also during a maximum straining effort so that any prolapsing hemorrhoids can be demonstrated. Inspection should focus on the presence of:

Dermatitis: A local-anesthetic-containing cream is a common cause of dermatitis in patients with hemorrhoids. Often a nonspecific "inflammatory" skin reaction is seen secondary to over the counter skin preparations, suppositories, deodorants, talc powder, or antiseptic ointments.

Abnormal skin conditions: Examination of the perianal skin may reveal *psoriasis* (characteristic scaly plaques); *eczema* (patches of inflamed skin usually in association with similar areas on other parts of the body and a history of atopy); *Bowen's disease* (reddish intradermal plaque); *leukemia* (discolored skin thickening); *vitiligo and albinism* (depigmentation); *thinning and depigmentation* (application of steroid creams); *allergic reaction* (blistering); *Crohn's disease* (inflamed skin tags with ulcers or fissures); *squamous carcinoma* (characteristic heaped up ulcer margins); or *Condyloma acuminata* (anal warts).

Surface discharges: In cases of prolapsing hemorrhoids, mucus may be present from irritation of the columnar mucosa above the dentate line. Both mucus and pus can be seen in patients with an anoglandular fistula, inflammatory bowel disease, gonorrhea, syphilis, or chlamydia.

Skin tags: A single skin tag is of little significance but multiple tags usually indicate underlying hemorrhoids, often large. They may be remnants of thrombosed external hemorrhoids in the past. Large, bulky, and swollen skin tags may also be associated with inflammatory bowel disease.

Hemorrhoids: A hemorrhoid is seen as a bluish-red cushion of prolapsing tissue at the anal orifice. A hemorrhoid visualized during inspection, especially if it is seen without straining, indicates that it is large and either third- or fourth-degree. A strangulated prolapsed internal-external hemorrhoid is visible as a bluish purple, tensely swollen, and tender lump protruding from the anal canal. A thrombosed external hemorrhoid is seen as a rounded, tensely swollen, smaller lump at the anal verge which does not extend above the dentate line.

Mucosa: Mucosa protruding from the anal orifice may be related to prolapsing internal hemorrhoids but can also be due to an anterior rectocele, ectropion, or a mucosal or full-thickness prolapse.

Rectal prolapse: Mucosal rectal prolapse is seen as irritated reddish mucosa at the anal verge. Most often it is circumferential but may be located in one quadrant only. Full thickness rectal prolapse is noted as bulky rectal tissue with circumferential ridges. The overlying mucosa may be irritated, bruised, or ulcerated. Prolapse is best visualized while the patient is seated on a commode and asked to strain.

Anorectal tumors: Squamous cell carcinoma presents as a painful ulcerated lesion. It causes bleeding, discharge, and itching. It is often confused with hemorrhoids by patients, leading to lethal consequences. Occasionally rectal cancers or polyps can protrude through the anal orifice and present outside. Melanoma appears as a painful lump which may or may not be pigmented. Therefore it can easily be confused with benign anorectal conditions and the diagnosis is often delayed. It may ulcerate or bleed. The verrucous carcinoma, or the so-called Buschke-Lowenstein tumor, presents as a large, fungating, warty, cauliflower-like growth which has a characteristic appearance and is unlikely to be missed by the examining physician.

Fissures: The external end of an anal fissure may be seen upon gently parting the buttocks. Occasionally, fissures are associated with hemorrhoids; but if multiple fissures are seen, especially if located laterally or anteriorly, they should raise the suspicion of Crohn's disease.

Sinuses or fistulas: Anoglandular fistulas may be seen. Rarely, fistulas may be secondary to Crohn's disease, tuberculosis, or cancer. The presence of discharge, the location of the opening, and its relationship to the hemorrhoids should be noted.

Anorectal varices: Large dilated veins may be seen at the anal verge communicating with the internal rectal varicosities.

Sphincter tone: A tightly closed anus may indicate spasm secondary to an anal fissure. A patulous anus may be caused by rectal prolapse or anal intercourse. Poor anal tone should caution the surgeon, as a hemorrhoidectomy in these patients may lead to fecal incontinence.

It is important to diligently and carefully look for and identify the above conditions, as they heavily impact upon the treatment of hemorrhoids. Many of these conditions will require treatment in their own right (fistulas, cancer). Most will complicate the proposed treatment of hemorrhoids (fecal incontinence, Crohn's disease). Some can be treated alongside any treatment of hemorrhoids (skin tags, fissures). In addition, an attempt should be made to clean up the diseased or excoriated perianal skin before hemorrhoidectomy. Any ulcerating lesion should be biopsied. A prolapsing "hemorrhoid" in a juvenile should initiate investigations to exclude a prolapsing polyp. A prolapsing "hemorrhoid" in an older patient should result in placing the patient on a commode where a circumferential rectal prolapse can be excluded. Treating hemorrhoids without attention to these details will invariably result in an unsatisfied patient.

In most cases, hemorrhoids are easily and instantly recognized by their typical appearance. A hemorrhoid is a bluish-red cushion of tissue covered by smooth, shiny mucosa. First-degree hemorrhoids are only visible by anoscopy, but larger hemorrhoids protrude to a greater or lesser extent through the external anal orifice. Straining increases the engorgement and prolapse of hemorrhoids. The apex, or the pedicle, which is located towards the rectum, is narrow and pink or red. The base, which tends to hang out, is broader and is bluish or purple. Skin tags may be located at this end.

Hemorrhoids occur most prominently in the left lateral (three o'clock), right posterior (seven o'clock) and right anterior (eleven o'clock) positions. When large, they hang out as radial folds in these three locations. When a circumferential prolapse of hemorrhoids is present, it may be difficult to differentiate from rectal prolapse. However, it should be emphasized that prolapsing hemorrhoids have radial folds with intervening grooves, as opposed to rectal prolapses which have circumferential folds.

Hemorrhoids that become complicated by thrombosis of the external anal venous network (below the dentate line) appear as a hard bluish-black lump in the perianal area. If untreated, the overlying epithelium is eroded by pressure necrosis and the blood clot starts protruding from the lump. Once the clot falls off, it leaves a small ulcer, which can mimic an ulcerating anal carcinoma. Hemorrhoids that become complicated by thrombosis of the prolapsed internal (and sometimes external) venous network cause severe pain. These strangulated piles require emergency treatment. The appearance of the tensely swollen black-bluish mass of tissue at the anal orifice, along with exquisite tenderness, is unmistakable. There is extensive edema and congestion of both external and internal hemorrhoids. If left untreated, the edema progresses to ulceration and necrosis.

It is important to emphasize that in every case of anorectal disease, visual inspection needs to be done twice: once with the patient relaxed and again with the patient making a straining effort. During straining, lesions that are otherwise hidden in the anal canal descend into view

(e.g., a polyp, hypertrophied anal papilla, mucosal prolapse). In the case of hemorrhoids, they may prolapse, thus placing them in a different category which may require another form of treatment. Important differential diagnoses such as mucosal or full-thickness rectal prolapse may become evident and any reduction in anal tone may become apparent, e.g., by a gaping response.

In summary, at the end of the visual inspection the proctologist should have identified not only the presence of any external or prolapsing internal hemorrhoids but also should have formed, together with the history, a shrewd assessment of the degree of the hemorrhoidal mass that is present. Providing no other complicating factors are encountered, it is usually possible at this stage to form a judgment on the likely treatment for this patient. It is a good principle to discuss these with the patient before any further examination or instrumentation is undertaken. Another opportunity may arise after proctoscopy, but verbal consent to any instrumentation, and especially to invasive treatment, must be obtained before further evaluation and treatment is undertaken.

Digital Examination

While the old aphorism "if you don't put your finger in it (anus), you might put your foot in it" is the best piece of advice for any student of medicine, it may not be so important in the diagnosis of hemorrhoids. It is difficult to feel uncomplicated hemorrhoids with a digital exam. This is because hemorrhoids are soft vascular cushions which will empty out and collapse easily under pressure of the examining finger.

With the patient in left lateral position and after appropriate warning, a well lubricated finger should be inserted into the anal canal. It is important to stroke the anus with the lubricated finger a few times before actually inserting the finger, as it will not only reassure the patient that the examiner is proceeding gently but also allow the anus to relax and open up a little. During this time, conversation is continued, as it will help the patient relax and take his mind off the examination.

Any suggestion of excessive pain should immediately deter the physician from proceeding any further. In this situation, an exam under sedation is warranted. It is unfortunate to see that so many physicians eagerly persist with a full digital rectal exam while their patients are in agonizing pain and screaming for mercy. I have also seen many patients with excruciatingly painful anal fissures or thrombosed hemorrhoids who have informed me that their physicians have made the diagnosis after performing an anoscopic examination in their office! I shudder to think of the agonizing pain inflicted on these poor souls. Such brutal practices of inserting a cold metallic object, or for that matter, even an index finger, in an acutely tender anus should be relegated to the past. These practices may have been appropriate in the torture dungeons of the Middle Ages but are not appropriate for a doctor's office. Any patient with a painful anorectal condition should be examined with the utmost gentle care to avoid any unnecessary discomfort. Such an exam will not only reassure the patient but is also helpful in establishing a trusting relationship between the proctologist and his patient.

Once the finger is in the anal canal, it should be rotated so that all quadrants can be examined. Not only should the lining mucosa be examined circumferentially, but the prostate, cervix, and other structures outside the rectum should be examined as well. The levator should be palpated to elicit any tenderness, and the dentate line should be felt for hypertrophied anal papillae. The patient is asked to contract the sphincters and the muscle tone is evaluated.

With the finger fully inserted, the patient is asked to strain, which may bring down pathology, such as a carcinoma, even from the upper rectum to the finger tip. As the finger is removed the patient is asked to strain down again. This may cause hemorrhoids or other polypoidal lesions to follow the finger as it is slowly withdrawn out of the anal canal. After removal, the finger is examined for any telltale sign of blood, mucus, or pus which may be indicative of another pathology. The proctologist will also have learned whether the rectum is loaded with feces, which may require an enema before proceeding further. If one is required, it should be given at this stage and the patient should be asked to proceed to the rest room.

Proctoscopy

After digital examination, the surgeon proceeds immediately with the visual examination of the rectum using a lighted proctoscope. Most colorectal surgeons use a rigid instrument, though flexible scopes are also being used increasingly. Proctoscopy (rigid sigmoidoscopy) does not require a routine bowel preparation. Most of the patients will have such sparse fecal contamination of their rectum that it does not interfere with a complete examination. Some will have small solid boluses of stools that can be maneuvered out of the way. Others will have liquid residues that can be evacuated with a large bore suction tube. Only a few patients will require a bowel preparation. As discussed earlier, bowel preparation not only imposes delay, with additional pressure on staff and toilet facilities, but can also result in loss of diagnostic information such as blood or pus from the rectum. In some patients, the preparation can also cause irritation and reddening of rectal mucosa which can be mistaken by the observer for proctitis.

Rigid proctoscopy requires that the instrument is passed through the rectosigmoid junction into the lower sigmoid colon, that is, to a full 25 cm from the anal verge. Unless this is done, the examination is diagnostically incomplete. Disposable plastic proctoscopes are now available which are not only inexpensive and safe but also improve visualization and examination (Fig. 4.2). These usually have a diameter of 19–20 mm. The small bore proctoscopes make it easier to get past fecal boluses and navigate around the haustral folds or areas of pathological narrowing. If needed, diagnostic maneuvers such as biopsy or polypectomy can also be performed through these scopes. Most importantly, they are more comfortable for patients.

The insertion of the proctoscope should be slow and gentle. The surgeon should talk to the patient and explain the procedure as the examination proceeds. With the obturator in place, and held in place by the thumb, the proctoscope is inserted into the anal canal. It should be advanced and directed towards the umbilicus first. Once the

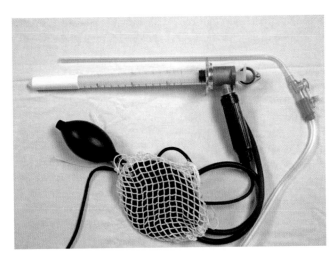

Figure 4.2 Proctoscope.

puborectalis sling is passed (about 3–4 cm from the anal verge), the proctoscope should be directed posteriorly into the hollow of the sacrum. The obturator is removed and the proctoscope is advanced under direct visualization. The valves of Houston are navigated and the scope is advanced along the sacral curve to the rectosigmoid junction. There may be another angulation here and it is often necessary to tilt the scope handle superiorly as it is navigated into the sigmoid colon, which is located inferiorly and to the left in a patient lying in the left lateral position.

The examination should be slow and gentle and accompanied by minimal insufflation of air. This helps in avoiding discomfort and reduces the small chance of accidental perforation of the rectum. During withdrawal, the scope is pulled back slowly and rotated circumferentially in a clockwise fashion to ensure complete visualization of all the walls of the rectum. Immediately before withdrawal, the viewing glass door should be opened to let out air and thereby minimize gas cramps.

Although the diagnosis of hemorrhoids is not made by the use of the proctoscope, every case of suspected hemorrhoids requires at least a complete examination of the rectum and distal sigmoid as an integral part of the workup. Anyone who has practiced long enough has seen those unfortunate cases where a "hemorrhoid" was being treated while a more sinister carcinoma was lurking in the proximal rectum. The complete examination of the rectum and lower sigmoid in patients with rectal bleeding cannot be overemphasized.

Flexible Sigmoidoscopy

Though rigid proctoscopy remains the instrument of choice in most coloproctology units, the flexible scope is being increasingly used in some clinics. The instrument is 60 cm in length and allows the surgeon to examine the colon up to the splenic flexure. Therefore its use requires bowel preparation, whose disadvantages have been alluded to earlier. The advantages of a flexible sigmoidoscope are: (a) It is less painful than rigid scopes. (b) It can reach up to the splenic flexure, thereby improving the yield of the examination. (c) It is easier to pass through the rectosigmoid junction.

The disadvantages of a flexible sigmoidoscope include: (a) The instrument is expensive and not readily available in most coloproctology offices. (b) Extra training and personnel are required. (c) Special cleaning methods and expensive cleaning machines are required. (d) Operative procedures are more limited. (e) Examination of the distal rectum, especially just above the anorectal junction is often unsatisfactory. (f) Bowel preparation is required. (g) Retained fecal matter in the rectum is more difficult to remove than with the large bore rigid proctoscope.

The individual colorectal surgeon must weigh the advantages and disadvantages of the flexible sigmoidoscope with regard to the demands of his individual practice style and requirements. Both rigid proctoscopes and flexible sigmoidoscopes have their advantages and disadvantages. Whatever method is used, the proctologist and staff should be well versed in its use and cleaning requirements. A routine should be developed and adhered to at all times.

Colonoscopy

A complete colonoscopy should be performed in all patients with unusual symptoms or in whom it is hard to attribute all the symptoms to hemorrhoids. These include patients with hemorrhoids who have altered bowel habits, abdominal cramps, a change in caliber of stools, the presence of mucus or pus in stools, weight loss, anemia, or a family history of colon cancer or polyps.

Patients in whom rectal bleeding is suspected to be from hemorrhoids, but who are more than 50 years old and have not had their screening endoscopy yet, should also undergo colonoscopy before treatment of hemorrhoids. This age limit should be reduced to 40 in patients who have a family history of colon cancer or polyps. In patients with a family history of polyposis syndromes or with a family history of carcinoma at an early age, the threshold for colonoscopy can be reduced to an even earlier age. Patients with iron deficiency anemia or a

positive fecal occult blood test should also undergo colonoscopy irrespective of age [4].

Anoscopy

Anoscopy is the examination of the anal canal. It should be done after visual and digital examination is completed. Also, because anoscopy is often accompanied by definitive treatment of the hemorrhoids, it should be done after proctoscopy has been completed. Therefore, it is considered the last and final part of the patient's examination. Needless to say, before performing this exam a formal or informal consent should have been obtained about any anticipated treatment plans or intervention.

A variety of anoscopes are available for use (Fig. 4.3). A Vernon-David anoscope is ideal for anorectal examination. It is not quite as large as a standard anoscope, which stretches the anal canal and hence results in an underestimation of the hemorrhoid size. In patients with deep cheeks of buttocks or long anal canals, most of whom are likely to be obese males, the longer and thinner Hinkel-James anoscope is preferred. Disposable clear plastic anoscopes are also available. Some anoscopes can be attached to a light source. In other cases, a head lamp can be worn by the examiner.

Whatever instrument is used, it should be tapered, with a diameter not to exceed 20–30 mm. It should have either an angled end or a longitudinal groove. I prefer the longitudinal groove because it allows the hemorrhoidal complex to protrude into the longitudinal slot and makes it accessible for the planned treatment.

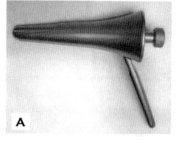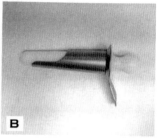

Figure 4.3 (A) Hinkel-James anoscope (B) Vernon-David anoscope.

A generous amount of lubrication should be used. The anoscope is gently and gradually inserted with its obturator. As the instrument is inserted, the perianal skin is gently teased or stretched with a finger to assist advancement. Only when the anoscope has been inserted to the fullest extent should the obturator be removed. Occasionally, there is a sudden gush of flatus or stools as the obturator is removed and the proctologist should be prepared for this. Any pain during insertion of the anoscope should raise the possibility of another pathology and mandate an examination under sedation. There is no point in persisting with an examination if the patient is experiencing pain as a result of the procedure.

Using the anoscope, every aspect of the anal canal is inspected. Normal as well as abnormal structures are noted. The identification of the pale, wavy dentate line is especially important because it separates the insensitive columnar mucosa above from the sensitive squamous epithelium below—a point of vital importance for many office procedures. With the anoscope in position, the patient is asked to strain so that the amount of prolapse can be assessed.

Certain conditions which commonly accompany hemorrhoids can be identified during anoscopy and proctoscopy and may modify treatment. These include: (a) *Fistula in ano:* This may present as a purulent discharge from the level of the dentate line. Treatment of the fistula takes precedence. (b) *Anal fissure:* Usually this would already have been identified during the history and visual inspection. However, some cases may be painless, and the proctologist may be surprised by an innocuous looking fissure in the anal canal along with the hemorrhoids. It is mandatory to proceed with a full examination under anesthesia in these cases to rule out either Crohn's disease or a carcinoma. If it does turn out to be a simple anal fissure then it can be treated in the same operation along with the hemorrhoids. (c) *Anal Condyloma:* Occasionally these may be found during anoscopy, without any perianal involvement. They can be fulgurated along with the treatment for hemorrhoids. (d) *Hypertrophied anal papilla:* A fibrotic tag at the entrance of the anal crypt at the dentate line can be excised at the same time as the hemorrhoids are treated. (e) *Proctitis:* This

may be simple inflammation (nonspecific proctitis); ulcerative (ulcerative colitis or Crohn's disease) or profusely productive (gonorrhea, chlamydia). (f) *Anorectal varices* are uncommon and can be seen in patients with portal hypertension. Extreme caution should be exercised in the treatment of "hemorrhoids" in these patients.

Once the diagnosis of hemorrhoids is confirmed upon anoscopy, an assessment should be made about their size, position, and number. At this stage an educated decision can be made about the best possible treatment. If they are suitable for immediate treatment and the patient has already been informed and agrees, the appropriate treatment (either banding or injection) can be initiated simultaneously.

Summary

As is true for all diseases, a firm and correct diagnosis must precede treatment. The diagnosis of hemorrhoids is made by taking a proper history followed by a complete examination. Examination includes visual inspection, digital rectal examination, proctoscopy, and anoscopy, in that order. Diagnosis is made not only by making a positive identification of hemorrhoids but also by ruling out alternative or additional conditions which may be present. This is achieved by a complete examination of the anal canal, rectum, and lower sigmoid. Unless this is done religiously in all cases, misdiagnosis is possible, sometimes with serious and occasionally with tragic consequences. If undue time appears to have been spent on the diagnosis of hemorrhoids in this chapter, it is because the consequences of misdiagnosis are severe and possibly lethal.

At the conclusion of the diagnostic assessment, both the presence and size of the hemorrhoids are known and a treatment plan can be determined. Provided the patient has already been informed, examination will seamlessly lead to the office treatment of smaller hemorrhoids, which can be performed at the conclusion of anoscopy.

References

1. Cataldo P, Ellis N, Gregorcyk S et al. Practice parameters for the management of hemorrhoids. Dis Colon Rectum 2005;48:189–94.
2. Nivatvongs S. Hemorrhoids. In: Gordon PH, Novatvongs S, eds. Principles and practice of surgery for the colon, rectum and anus. Quality Medical Publishing Inc. 1999:193–215.
3. Smith LE. Hemorrhoids. In: Fazio VW, Church JM, Delaney CP, eds. Current therapy in colon and rectal surgery. Elsevier Mosby, 2004:11–22.
4. Rex DK, Bond JH, Winawer S et al. Quality in the technical performance of colonoscopy and the continuous quality improvement process for colonoscopy: Recommendations of the US Multi-Society Task Force on Colorectal Cancer. Am J Gastroenterol 2002;97:1296–308.

5 Indications for Intervention

Khawaja Azimuddin

Most patients with hemorrhoids present with painless bright red bleeding. However, the diagnosis should never be assumed and should be arrived at only after a thorough and detailed history and physical examination as outlined in the chapter on diagnosis. "Diagnosis must precede any treatment," is an important surgical dictum which is occasionally forgotten in the heat of events, often with tragic consequences.

Provided that the diagnosis is confirmed, the next challenge is to identify the severity of the patient's symptoms. The treatment must be tailored to the patient's problems. Certainly, it would be most inappropriate to perform a painful excisional hemorrhoidectomy in a patient who has an occasional asymptomatic prolapse and is otherwise not incapacitated by the disease. Since vascular anal cushions are a normal part of the anatomy, the term "hemorrhoids" should be confined to situations where these cushions are abnormally large and cause symptoms. In the absence of symptoms, even very large cushions do not require treatment. The old adage that it is hard to make an asymptomatic patient better applies here.

A variety of treatment options are available for the treatment of hemorrhoids. Proper attention must be made in the selection of cases for any treatment options that are available. The selection depends upon the degree of discomfort that the patient is experiencing as well as an accurate assessment of the size and bulk of the hemorrhoids. Not every patient with hemorrhoids

requires surgical intervention. Often patients with hemorrhoids suffer from minor symptoms which are inconvenient and unpleasant at most. A surgical hemorrhoidectomy in these patients would most certainly be an overtreatment. It would be akin to treating a fungal toe infection with an amputation!

It is also important to understand the patient's expectations. Many patients who have mild symptoms are looking for reassurance that there is nothing more sinister going on. Once the evaluation is complete and other causes have been ruled out, these patients may not be interested in surgical intervention and can just be treated with education about healthy eating habits and good bowel habits. Common indications for intervention in patients with hemorrhoids include bleeding and prolapse. Other indications are mucus seepage and pruritis, fecal soiling and incontinence, pain and thrombosis, and anemia. These, along with some special situations, will be discussed individually.

Bleeding

Bleeding is the most common indication for intervention in patients with hemorrhoids. The first priority is to rule out other more important sources of rectal bleeding. Once the diagnosis is confirmed, a treatment plan should be

I. Khubchandani et al. (eds.), *Surgical Treatment of Hemorrhoids*, DOI 10.1007/978-1-84800-314-9_5,
© Springer-Verlag London Limited 2009

devised which would be appropriate for the patient's symptoms.

Bleeding without prolapse occurs in small (first-degree) internal hemorrhoids. These small hemorrhoids do not require surgical treatment. Most often the symptoms can be controlled by correcting the factors which cause the hemorrhoids to bleed, such as hard stools, straining at defecation, lack of exercise, and faulty eating habits. Patients should be advised about eating a high fiber diet, increasing the intake of water, and avoiding straining during defecation [1]. Fiber supplements such as Metamucil®, Fibercon®, Konsyl®, or Citrucel® are very useful and may completely stop the bleeding.

Occasionally, antihemorrhoidal suppositories such as Anusol® are useful, but I am not a fan of these remedies. If bleeding persists or becomes worse, infrared coagulation or sclerotherapy may be offered, as will be discussed in other chapters. Since hemorrhoids are rarely cured by nonoperative treatments, follow-up is always advisable.

Bleeding with prolapse that reduces spontaneously (second-degree hemorrhoids) is most often treated with rubber band ligation. Bleeding in conjunction with hemorrhoids that prolapse and have to be reduced manually (third-degree), usually requires multiple episodes of banding, multiple suture ligation, or the procedure for prolapse and hemorrhoids (PPH). As hemorrhoids enlarge, they remain prolapsed and cannot be reduced. Such large (fourth-degree) hemorrhoids most often require surgical excision [2]. These treatments and their indications will be discussed separately in the ensuing chapters.

In some patients with painless rectal bleeding, anoscopy and proctoscopy in the office does not confirm the clinical suspicion of hemorrhoids. In such cases there should be no reluctance in arranging a full colonoscopy and even an anorectal exam under anesthesia. A hemorrhoid or an alternate diagnosis may be unearthed during such an exam in the operating room. The consequences of missing a tumor are devastating, and one must not hesitate to do a full exam even in a young patient.

Prolapse

Prolapse is another common symptom of hemorrhoids. Most patients with prolapse will suffer from bleeding, dragging discomfort, mucus discharge, and pruritis. Intervention is offered to alleviate these symptoms. Just as with bleeding, prolapse by itself is not an indication for intervention unless it is symptomatic. However, as prolapse is indicative of the increasing size of the hemorrhoidal plexus, it is invariably associated with the above symptoms. Usually the larger the hemorrhoidal complex and the more the prolapse, the worse are the symptoms. Not all patients with large hemorrhoids will have unbearable symptoms. Conversely some patients with small hemorrhoids will experience annoying symptoms. Therefore, the size of the hemorrhoid does not always correlate with the symptoms and size is not considered to be a reliable indicator for intervention.

Occasionally a patient with large perpetually prolapsed hemorrhoids will become so accustomed to their presence that he is not unduly disturbed. In these patients, the surface mucosa becomes calloused and they hardly bleed or secrete mucus. The surgeon should not impose a hemorrhoidectomy on such patients, especially if they are reluctant and are not having any pain. Sometimes these patients are completely asymptomatic except for the prolapse. Often reassurance, after a thorough examination, is all that these patients are looking for. It should be clear from the above discussion that the recommendation for surgery is based on symptoms rather than on the size of the hemorrhoids.

If the extent of prolapse is slight and reduces spontaneously (second-degree), it may well respond to nonoperative treatment. Sclerotherapy or infrared coagulation are excellent techniques, although several treatment sessions are usually required to produce worthwhile shrinkage of the prolapsing tissue. In my opinion, rubber banding is more effective for these second-degree hemorrhoids.

In patients with third-degree hemorrhoids that prolapse but can be reduced manually, an

Table 5.1. Stages of Hemorrhoids and Recommended Treatments

Stage	Definition	Treatment
I	Bleeding, no prolapse	High fiber diet
II	Prolapse reduces spontaneously	Fixation/destruction (IRC, RBL, sclerotherapy)
III	Prolapse that is manually reducible	Fixation/destruction (PPH, RBL, suture ligation)
IV	Prolapse that cannot be reduced	Fixation/destruction (PPH, hemorrhoidectomy)

IRC: infrared coagulation. RBL: rubber band ligation. PPH: procedure for prolapse and hemorrhoids.

anopexy (i.e., "procedure for prolapse of hemorrhoids" or PPH) is most often performed. These hemorrhoids can also be treated with multiple episodes of rubber banding in the office if the patient is unwilling or unfit (by way of medical comorbidities) to undergo an operation. Another option is to shrink down the vascular tissue by performing either a "blind" or ultrasound-directed suture ligation in multiple areas. Some of these hemorrhoids are large and fleshy and cause significant symptoms, and the proctologist may be justified in offering a hemorrhoidectomy in selected patients. For large symptomatic permanently prolapsed fourth-degree internal/external hemorrhoids, an excisional hemorrhoidectomy is the procedure of choice [3]. Rarely, an anopexy or PPH may be performed. The treatment plan is summarized in Table 5.1.

Mucus and Pruritis

Hemorrhoids can cause seepage of mucus from the anal canal. It is secondary to overproduction of mucus by a chronically prolapsed and irritated hemorrhoid. Occasionally, very large and bulky hemorrhoidal cushions prevent proper sealing of the anal orifice and predispose to leakage of mucus. Treatment of hemorrhoids in these groups of patients is justifiable for relief of symptoms. Excessive mucus may be produced in patients with inflammatory bowel disease, nonspecific proctitis, villous adenoma, carcinoma, or rectal prolapse. Only when these other sources of mucus overproduction have been ruled out, should treatment of hemorrhoids for pruritis and mucus seepage be carried out.

Mucus leakage is a common cause of pruritis ani. Irritation of the perianal skin from the protein-rich mucus produces burning and itching. The perianal skin may become macerated, soggy, and excoriated. These symptoms are usually associated with large internal hemorrhoids, and surgical treatment is certainly indicated in this group of patients. In cases where the cause is an incompetent anal sphincter rather than hemorrhoids, a high fiber diet, Kegel exercises, and placement of a cotton pledget at the anal orifice will often suffice. If there is no evidence of another cause of reduced sphincter tone and large hemorrhoids are confirmed, a hemorrhoidectomy can be advised even if symptoms of mucus/pruritis cannot be unequivocally linked to the hemorrhoids. However, before resorting to such surgery, it must be ensured that the patient does have large hemorrhoids and that he understands that success is not guaranteed.

Pruritis can also result from inadequate cleaning after bowel movements because of large skin tags. These skin tags allow the fecal debris to hide under the skin folds and cause irritation and maceration of the perianal skin. Hemorrhoidectomy with excision of skin tags will resolve this problem.

Long standing mucus leakage is often associated with excoriation and dermatitis of the perianal skin. Before embarking upon an excisional hemorrhoidectomy, all efforts must be made to treat the dermatitis, because a soggy and inflamed skin will slow down postoperative healing. Protective skin barriers and warm sitz baths will immensely help to achieve this goal and should be started before surgical intervention.

Fecal Soiling and Incontinence

Fecal soiling and minor incontinence problems are occasionally associated with hemorrhoids. Large chronically prolapsed hemorrhoids may cause incomplete closure of the anal canal and predispose to mucus and fecal leakage. Such patients will complain of minor incontinence problems. On the other hand, a hemorrhoidectomy in itself may cause occult fecal incontinence to manifest.

The anal canal is kept closed during rest by the action of sphincter muscles. Once the internal sphincter is tightly contracted, there is still a small hole left in the anal canal. The soft vascular hemorrhoidal cushions act as a plug to fill in this small gap and help maintain continence. A hemorrhoidectomy, by removing these cushions, may contribute to incontinence. Therefore, a previously unrecognized sphincter injury from childbirth, internal sphincterotomy, or fistulotomy may manifest after a surgical hemorrhoidectomy because the vascular cushion/plug is lost. There may also be undocumented sphincter injury during hemorrhoidectomy from the insertion of large retractors or the now abandoned Lord's dilation, which routinely preceded hemorrhoidectomy in the past. It is therefore important to establish the presence and degree of fecal incontinence before embarking upon the surgical treatment of hemorrhoids.

Frank fecal incontinence should never be attributed to hemorrhoids, as the cause is invariably elsewhere. Hemorrhoidectomy will only make matters worse in these cases. An important cause of incontinence, which is often confused with hemorrhoids, is rectal prolapse. The proctologist should have a high index of suspicion when a patient with "prolapsing hemorrhoids" complains of incontinence. These patients should be examined on a commode, while straining, to rule out rectal prolapse.

Pain and Thrombosis

Uncomplicated hemorrhoids do not cause pain. A large prolapsed hemorrhoid can cause a dragging sensation; but in this case, the hemorrhoidectomy would most likely be offered because of the accompanying symptoms of prolapse, not because of pain. Anorectal pain may be due to other concomitant conditions, such as a fissure or fistula. In the case of an anal fissure, it can be treated at the time of surgery for hemorrhoids. When dealing with large fourth-degree hemorrhoids, they can be excised and an open partial internal sphincterotomy can be performed at the same time. On the other hand, if the hemorrhoids are small, they can be suture ligated and a submucosal internal sphincterotomy can be performed at the same time.

In patients with an anal fistula and hemorrhoids, both conditions can be treated surgically at the same time. The hemorrhoids can be ligated or excised, if away from the fistulotomy wound. Since the hemorrhoidal cushions normally assist in closing the anal canal and maintaining continence, caution should be exercised in removing large bulks of tissue in order to avoid postoperative incontinence.

Perhaps there is no other more compelling indication for hemorrhoidectomy than an acutely painful thrombosed internal/external hemorrhoid. Internal hemorrhoids which are complicated by thrombosis cause severe acute pain. The prolapsed hemorrhoid becomes trapped outside the anal canal by spasm of the sphincter muscles and cannot be reduced. It soon loses its blood supply and becomes strangulated. The appearance of the exquisitely tender, tensely swollen, bluish-black mass of edematous tissue protruding from the anal orifice is unmistakable. Most of these patients have a history of long-standing hemorrhoidal disease. Proper treatment requires emergency or urgent hemorrhoidectomy in the operating room.

A thrombosed external hemorrhoid, on the other hand, is a self-limiting condition. If the patient is seen within 72 hours and is still having acute pain, excision should be offered [1]. This can easily be done in the office under local anesthesia. If the patient is seen after 72 hours, or when the acute pain and swelling is already resolving, it may be best left alone. Conservative management with sitz baths, nonconstipating analgesics, and bulk-producing agents is recommended, and the condition will spontaneously resolve.

Anemia

Very rarely anemia can be caused by bleeding hemorrhoids. Before embarking upon treatment of hemorrhoids, all other sources of anemia, such as malignancy, occult gastrointestinal loss, excessive menstrual loss, or inflammatory bowel disease should be ruled out. Hemorrhoids must never be blamed for anemia until a thorough and systemic examination of the entire body has been completed and all other causes have been ruled out. A full GI evaluation and colonoscopy must precede treatment. The treatment offered will depend on the staging of the hemorrhoids.

Special Circumstances

Associated Anorectal Conditions

Patients with symptomatic hemorrhoids who also have associated benign anorectal conditions may undergo surgery to deal with both issues at the same time. Occasionally the choice of operation is influenced by the coexisting benign condition. Patients who have large symptomatic skin tags may undergo excisional hemorrhoidectomy. However, excision should be conservative. Complete removal of the skin tags should never be the goal of the surgery, because it may lead not only to excessive pain but also to anal stenosis. A hypertrophied anal papilla can be excised at the same time as hemorrhoidectomy or suture ligation.

Patients who have hemorrhoids and anal fistulas can undergo ligation or excision of the hemorrhoids at the time of fistulotomy. An anal fissure associated with large third- or fourth-degree hemorrhoids can be treated with partial internal sphincterotomy during the hemorrhoidectomy. A fissure associated with smaller hemorrhoids can be treated with submucosal internal sphincterotomy while the hemorrhoids are suture ligated.

Pregnancy, Labor, and Delivery

Pregnancy and childbirth is the prime cause of hemorrhoids in young females. The hormonal milieu of pregnancy, increased pelvic blood flow, and the increased pelvic pressure in late pregnancy and delivery contribute to the development of hemorrhoids. Furthermore, there is a tendency towards constipation and straining during pregnancy and delivery, and this will also aggravate hemorrhoids. Once pregnancy is over, the hemorrhoids tend to improve over the next few months. Therefore, there is no need to rush into surgery in this group of patients.

However, as with all other patients, pregnant females with rectal bleeding must be evaluated by proctoscopy. The literature is full of cases where cancers and not hemorrhoids were the source of rectal bleeding in young pregnant females. There is literature supporting the idea that colorectal cancer in pregnant females grows faster because of the hormonal milieu, is more distally distributed, and is diagnosed at an advanced stage.

Hemorrhoidectomy is indicated during pregnancy only if acute prolapse and thrombosis occur [4]. It can be performed under local anesthesia in the lithotomy or left lateral position. If thrombosis occurs during delivery, a hemorrhoidectomy can be performed in the immediate postpartum period.

Anorectal Varices

Patients with portal hypertension may have anorectal varices. However, the incidence of hemorrhoids in patients with portal hypertension is no greater than in the normal population [5]. Although uncommon, massive bleeding may occur from hemorrhoids in patients with portal hypertension. Most commonly, it is seen during treatment of encephalopathy when the patient is receiving medications such as lactulose, neomycin, and potassium replacements, all of which may cause diarrhea and irritate the lining of the anal canal.

Attempts should be made to control the diarrhea, keep the stools soft and bulky, correct coagulopathy, and avoid rectal enemas or suppositories. If all else fails, the bleeding hemorrhoid can be ligated with a figure of eight suture. Hemorrhoidectomy should only be performed if suture ligation fails to control the bleeding.

Leukemia

Conservative management should always be attempted first. The risks of operative intervention include infection, poor wound healing, and bleeding from coexisting coagulopathy.

Inflammatory Bowel Disease

Indications for surgical treatment of hemorrhoids in patients with ulcerative colitis are no different than in any other patient population. In patients with Crohn's disease, hemorrhoidectomy is a relative contraindication. Complications of delayed wound healing, fissures, and fistulas have been reported. However, some authors have reported uncomplicated healing, especially when hemorrhoidectomy is performed in a quiescent stage [6]. A period of active management of IBD that includes rectal anti-inflammatory suppositories or enemas must precede surgery.

Bleeding Tendency

Patients who are on Coumadin, Plavix®, Aspirin, or other nonsteroidal anti-inflammatory drugs will have a tendency to bleed with even small hemorrhoids. In some patients these drugs cannot be stopped without serious consequences for the coronary or cerebral circulation. These patients should be treated with fiber supplements (Metamucil), increasing their intake of water and avoiding straining during defecation. If there is no improvement with the above measures, then surgical intervention may be required in patients with even small hemorrhoids.

Summary

Hemorrhoidal vascular cushions are a normal part of human anatomy. Therefore, hemorrhoids that are not causing any symptoms do not require treatment. The presence of even symptomatic hemorrhoids is not a life threatening illness and does not demand intervention. The purpose of any treatment of hemorrhoids is relief of symptoms rather than cure. Therefore, the treatment should not be worse than the disease itself.

In summary, bleeding without prolapse usually responds to nonoperative treatment. Prolapse may respond to banding, but may require surgery. Choice of the right procedure is decided principally by the size (degree) of the hemorrhoidal prolapse. Third-degree hemorrhoids are most often treated with PPH, whereas fourth-degree hemorrhoids will require excisional hemorrhoidectomy. Pain is not caused by uncomplicated hemorrhoids.

Thrombosis of external hemorrhoids can be managed by evacuation of the clot, whereas thrombosis of the internal hemorrhoids is best managed by immediate hemorrhoidectomy. However, if presentation is delayed and pain is already improving, conservative expectant management should be offered. Spontaneous resolution is the rule. Mucus leakage, pruritis, and fecal soiling may sometimes be associated with hemorrhoids, and these will be relieved by surgical intervention.

Providing a surgeon takes proper care that the indications for any of his treatments are proportional to the patient's symptoms, a successful result can be guaranteed. Careful analysis of both patient symptoms and patient expectations should be matched against the most effective modality of treatment for their relief.

References

1. Cataldo P, Ellis N, Gregorcyk S et al. Practice parameters for the management of hemorrhoids. Dis Colon Rectum 2005;48:189–94.
2. Smith LE. Hemorrhoids. In: Fazio VW, Church JM, Delaney CP, eds. Current therapy in colon and rectal surgery. Elsevier Mosby, 2004:11–22.

3. MacRae HM, McLeod RS. Comparison of hemorrhoidal treatment modalities: a meta-analysis. Dis Colon Rectum 1995;38:687–94.

4. Nivatvongs S. Hemorrhoids. In: Gordon PH, Novatvongs S, eds. Principles and practice of surgery for the colon, rectum and anus. Quality Medical Publishing Inc. 1999:193–215.

5. Hosking SW, Johnson AG, Smart HL et al. Anorectal varices, hemorrhoids, and portal hypertension. Lancet 1989;1:349–52.

6. Wolkomir AF, Lutchtefeld M. Surgery for symptomatic hemorrhoids and anal fissures in Crohn's disease. Dis Colon Rectum 1993;36:545–47.

6 Conservative/Nonoperative Therapy

Nina J. Paonessa

Introduction

Conservative therapy is used primarily for first-degree hemorrhoids but is also used in conjunction with other treatment modalities for all degrees of hemorrhoids. This is the primary form of treatment for the high risk patient as well. Conservative, nonoperative therapy centers on diet and behavior modifications. In addition, topical medications and suppositories may be used but the benefit is questionable. In summary, there are three mainstays of conservative management:

1. Bulking agents
2. Sitz baths/warm compresses
3. Local applications

Diet Modification/Stool Bulking Agents

The shearing effect caused by the hard stool or a sudden act of defecation as in urgent diarrhea, is thought to be responsible for the prolapse of the anal cushions [1]. The idea behind diet modification and stool bulking agents is to have a soft, formed stool which eliminates straining at defecation and thereby prevents prolapse of the anal cushions. Hard stools also cause hemorrhoids to bleed.

A diet which includes 20–30 g/day of fiber is recommended. This may be in the form of fruits and vegetables, raw, unprocessed wheat, oat bran, or psyllium seed. There are numerous over-the-counter fiber supplements available for those patients who cannot obtain enough fiber in their diets. These are in the form of tablets, powders, or wafers (see Table 6.1). Manufacturers have now made these colorless, tasteless, and even fruit-flavored. The main complaint with fiber supplements is abdominal bloating or cramping. In order to minimize these symptoms, patients are instructed to start at the lowest dose and gradually increase the dose to the desired effect, which is a soft, formed stool. Patients are also advised to drink plenty of water (at least 8–12 ounces/day). It is also important to educate patients that fiber supplements are effective over a period of time and do not work instantaneously. Patients should be advised to avoid constipating foods such as cheese/dairy products, chocolate, and caffeine.

Patients with diarrhea and hemorrhoidal symptoms should first have the etiology of the diarrhea investigated. Once this has been done, they should receive dietary manipulation with fiber and antidiarrheals as indicated [2]. The pruritus associated with hemorrhoids is also best treated with diet modification. Patients should be educated to avoid those foods that create an alkaline pH of the stool, thereby irritating the perianal area. These foods include: coffee, tea, cheese, chocolate, cola, citrus fruits and juices, beer, tomatoes, onions, and nuts.

I. Khubchandani et al. (eds.), *Surgical Treatment of Hemorrhoids*, DOI 10.1007/978-1-84800-314-9_6,
© Springer-Verlag London Limited 2009

Table 6.1 Common Brand-Name Fiber Supplements

Brand Name	Type of Fiber	Fiber Content
Konsyl® (Konsyl Pharmaceuticals)	psyllium	6 g/8 oz water
Fiber-Sure™ (Procter & Gamble)	inulin (vegetable fiber)	5 g/8 oz water
Metamucil® (Procter & Gamble)	psyllium husk	3.4 g/8 oz water
capsules,		
wafers,		
powder		
Benefiber® (Novartis)	wheat dextran	3 g/8 oz water
Citrucel®	methylcellulose	2 g/8 oz water
Citrucel Fibershake® (GlaxoSmith Kline)		

Sitz Baths

Sitz baths (soaking in a warm tub) are used to help soothe the uncomfortable perianal area and help reduce anal canal pressures. In some cases, baths also help in the manual reduction of prolapsed internal hemorrhoids by decreasing the swelling of the hemorrhoids and decreasing anal canal pressures. However, care must be taken to avoid prolonged soaking as this has the reverse effect and may cause perianal edema. For those patients who do not have access to a sitz bath or cannot get in and out of a bathtub, warm compresses may accomplish the same results.

Topical Agents

There are a multitude of suppositories, foams, and topical gels and ointments marketed for the treatment of hemorrhoids. None have been proven to "cure" hemorrhoids, but they may temporarily provide symptomatic relief. Topical hydrocortisone (e.g., Anusol®, ProctoFoam®) may reduce symptoms caused by pruritus; however, prolonged use may cause perianal skin attenuation and injury [2]. The ointments with an anesthetic (e.g., Analpram®, Lidocaine®) are beneficial only for pain relief for thrombosed external hemorrhoids.

References

1. Nivatvongs S. Hemorrhoids. In: Gordon PH, Nivatvongs S. (3rd ed). Principles and practice of surgery for the colon, rectum and anus. Quality Medical Publishing, Inc. 2007: 144–166.
2. Beck DE. Hemorrhoidal Disease. In: Beck DE, Wexner SD. (2nd ed). Fundamentals of anorectal surgery. Elsevier Science Limited 2002: 237–253.

7 Anal Dilation Treatment

P.H. Lord

Introduction

The theoretical background to the employment of dilatation for the treatment of haemorrhoids depends principally on the following precepts:

1) Haemorrhoids consist of loose connective tissue which contains thin-walled sinusoids fed with oxygenated blood via small arterioles. The sinusoids drain via vessels which run upwards in the submucosa of the lower rectum for at least three centimetres before they penetrate the muscular lamina propria to eventually link with the portal system (Fig. 7.1). While the draining vessels are in the submucosa they are easily obstructed by any raising of intrarectal or intra-abdominal pressure, causing backflow and rapid engorgement of the haemorrhoid plexus (Fig. 7.2). Much of our current understanding of the nature of haemorrhoids, and their relation to anal cushions – normal structures present from birth – stems from the work of W.H. Thomson.

2) That, in cases of haemorrhoids, a band (or bands) of fibrosis can be felt in the circular muscle of the anal sphincter and lower rectum. Attention to the existence of this band was originally drawn by Ernest Miles (1919) who named it the "pecten band", although he thought wrongly that the band lay in the subcutaneous tissue. As a consequence of the fibrous ring(s), even when the anal sphincter relaxes to allow stool to pass, the lumen remains restricted, thus generating higher intrarectal pressures.

3) Chronic persistent rise in pressure in the lower rectum and anal canal during defaecation causes permanent stretching and enlargement of the haemorrhoid veins and other supporting tissues, converting normal cushions to abnormal haemorrhoids. Straining habits of defaecation contribute an important element for back-pressure on the pelvic and haemorrhoidal veins, increasing the degree of engorgement.

4) Once the presence of a haemorrhoid is established, mechanical pressure, as when a hard constipated stool is squeezed through the constricted anal outlet, dislocates the pile in a downward direction, causing progressive problems of prolapse as well as aggravating venous engorgement of the anal veins.

One way to reverse the interlocking causes of increased ano-rectal pressure responsible for greater venous engorgement would be to permanently lower the element of outlet obstruction by stretching the fibrotic bands in the anal sphincter muscle. This is achieved by digital dilatation according to the method described below.

Indications

It is most important to stress that *elective dilatation is a treatment that is reserved for symptomatic haemorrhoids that would justify a haemorrhoidectomy* (i.e., third- and fourth-degree piles).

I. Khubchandani et al. (eds.), *Surgical Treatment of Hemorrhoids*, DOI 10.1007/978-1-84800-314-9_7,
© Springer-Verlag London Limited 2009

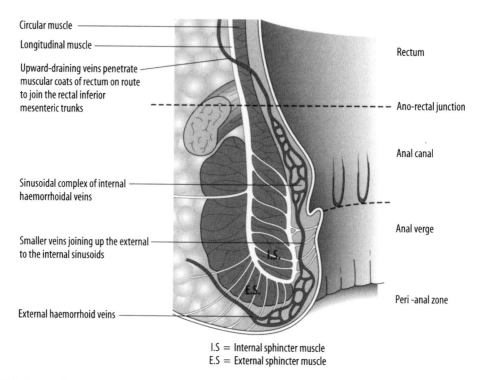

Circular muscle

Longitudinal muscle

Upward-draining veins penetrate
muscular coats of rectum on route
to join the rectal inferior
mesenteric trunks

Rectum

Ano-rectal junction

Anal canal

Sinusoidal complex of internal
haemorrhoidal veins

Anal verge

Smaller veins joining up the external
to the internal sinusoids

I.S.

E.S.

Peri-anal zone

External haemorrhoid veins

I.S = Internal sphincter muscle
E.S = External sphincter muscle

Figure 7.1. Note that the normal route of the blood draining from the haemorrhoidal venous sinusoids is upwards, and that the blood exits by penetrating the circular muscle coat of the rectum above the ano-rectal junction. The squeezing effect of **increased muscle tone** or a **constricting band** in the upper anal canal will cause back flow and engorgement of the veins of the anal cushions and haemorrhoids. Prevention of high anal sphincter tone or dilatation of any constricting ('pecten') bands will abolish the causes of abnormal venous engorgement. There are veins which connect the external and internal veins which can allow involvement of the external veins by engorgement factors which start in the internal (haemorrhoidal) veins.

The procedure can be used for the management of acute prolapsed thrombosed haemorrhoids ("strangulated piles") as described in Ch. 7.

Contraindications

Haemorrhoids which would not qualify for treatment by a haemorrhoidectomy are not suitable for treatment by dilatation.

First- and second-degree haemorrhoids should be treated by other methods (e.g., sclerotherapy, banding, or cryotherapy).

Asymptomatic haemorrhoids should not be treated by dilatation.

If the patient has large piles but the symptoms are not due to haemorrhoids but arise from another source (e.g., mucous leakage causing pruritus; mucosal prolapse), dilatation is contraindicated, not only because the symptoms will persist, but also because they may be worsened, after dilatation.

Patients with a weak sphincter should not undergo dilatation, not least because their prolapsing tissue will consist of ano-rectal mucosa rather than haemorrhoids (although associated haemorrhoids may well be present). Whenever mucosal prolapse is responsible for the symptoms rather than haemorrhoids, and most especially if a weak sphincter is the cause of the problem, a surgical answer is indicated (e.g., haemorrhoidectomy) although stapling may be used as an alternative (see Ch. 14).

No patient should undergo dilatation who has not passed through strict diagnostic procedures, which should include a careful history, expert examination, and procto-sigmoidoscopy plus

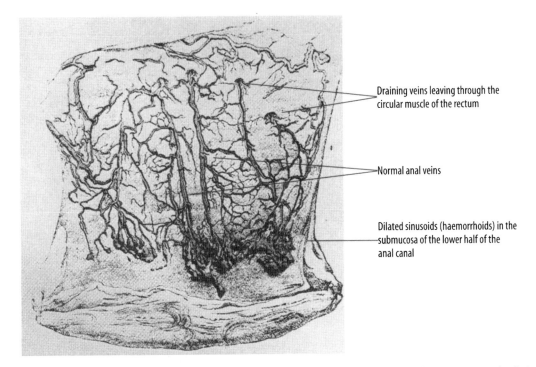

Draining veins leaving through the circular muscle of the rectum

Normal anal veins

Dilated sinusoids (haemorrhoids) in the submucosa of the lower half of the anal canal

Figure 7.2. After injection of the anal veins with a resin solution, the anal canal has been opened out and the overlying mucosa removed to display the veins. Note the dilated sinusoids in the lower half of the anal canal – the haemorrhoidal plexus.

colonoscopy and/or barium enema when necessary. The surgeon should have a low threshold for arranging a colonoscopy or barium enema (see Ch. 4: Diagnosis).

Technique

1. Preparation.
Provided due attention has been paid to correct diagnosis by examination of the patient, which must include a satisfactory (i.e., complete) sigmoidoscopy, no special preparation is required.

Informed consent should be obtained and signed for by the patient. Possible complications should be discussed, even if they are unlikely.

2. Anaesthesia.
A general anaesthetic is often used, and the anaesthetist should be experienced. The anaesthetist must take all necessary precautions to ensure that the patient is fit for anaesthesia. It helps if the surgeon and anaesthetist are accustomed to working as a team and have a pre-arranged system in place for carrying out the procedure.

A caudal block can be used as a very effective alternative to general anaesthesia, but takes more time, both pre- and post-operation. A caudal block can be a good choice for patients who are unsuitable for, or unwilling to undergo, a general anaesthetic.

Pre-medication is not required.

3. Position.
As the patient is fully conscious, positioning is easy. The patient is settled comfortably on the left side (left lateral position), with the knees drawn up and the buttocks projecting well over the edge of the table. Once the patient is in the correct position, the anaesthetic is commenced. Dilatation should not start until the anaesthetist is sure that the patient will not react to the dilatation in a dangerous way (e.g., by laryngeal spasm), as tracheal intubation is not employed.

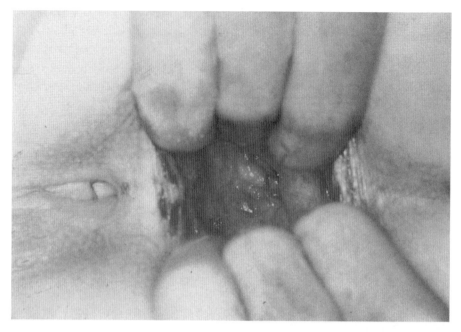

Figure 7.3. Note the following features. 1) That there is an unimpeded passage between the anal orifice and the rectum; the lumen of the latter is clearly seen. 2) That in this case, three fingers of each hand have been deemed sufficient for the dilatation. 3) That the fingers are only slightly curved, i.e., not hook-shaped. 4) That the anal mucosa and perianal skin are undamaged, i.e., that the dilatation has been gradual and gentle.

4. Dilation technique.

Standing at the patient's back, the surgeon ensures that the anus and his gloves are well lubricated. Two fingers of the left hand are inserted, and, with the digits partially hooked, they are lifted to open out the anal canal. The right index finger is now slipped in and pressed downwards, thus identifying all constricting bands. It must be remembered that some bands may be present as high as the fingers can reach.

Having ascertained the positions of all bands that are present (usually only one – the "Pecten Band"), the dilation can begin. This is usually done with the surgeon standing near to the bottom of the table. Only the two index fingers are used for initial dilation, and it is done with a gentle ironing out motion – like "ironing out the perineum when delivering a baby's head". *Care is taken not to damage the sphincter muscles.* Gradually the constricting bands are felt to give way. As the dilation proceeds, extra fingers are *fully* inserted as required to achieve the required end result, which should be abolition of all constrictions, leaving *an unobstructed passage from mid rectum to the exterior* such that even a well-formed stool could be extruded without any build-up of rectal pressures by straining (Fig. 7.3).

During the dilatation, the surgeon should remember that the anal sphincter is thinner and weaker at front and back and should concentrate stretching at the sides (i.e., 3 o'clock and 9 o'clock positions). *It is always better to do too little rather than too much.* If the dilatation is done gradually and gently, rather than abruptly and forcefully, sphincter muscle should be preserved from damage, and the anoderm should not be torn.

When the procedure is concluded, a decision is made as to whether insertion of a sponge is needed. A soft sponge can help to minimise post-stretch haematoma formation, but its removal (after the patient has woken up from the anaesthetic) can be the most unpleasant part of the procedure for the patient. Nor is there any evidence that its insertion makes any difference to the end results. The surgeon should make his own decision on use of a sponge as judged at the end of each dilatation.

Post-dilatation Care

Once the patient has recovered from the anaesthetic, and any sponges have been removed, they are allowed home. They are warned that defaecation may be a different experience, especially for the first few weeks. Straining should be abolished, and stool passage may be so effortless that it will occur quickly, almost without warning. In the early days after dilatation, incontinence may occur, especially on exertion, sneezing or straining; recovery from these initial effects can be speeded up by simple medications (e.g., codeine phosphate tablets) and sphincter exercises. Provided patients have been properly briefed on what to expect, and what action to take, they are able to manage any early problems without difficulty, and are happy to accept any temporary complications until normal control is re-established; a pad may be needed for the first few weeks until full control returns.

Once the patient has established normal post-dilatation defaecation, they are advised to add bran to their diet, along with plentiful fluids (see Ch. 6), to prevent recurrence of straining habits of defaecation and/or the hard stools that promoted their haemorrhoidal complaints in the first place.

If a patient continues to be troubled by prolapsing tissue (usually with mucosa as its principal component) this should be treated appropriately. In many cases, prolapsing mucosa can be treated effectively by banding (Ch. 9) or cryotherapy (Ch. 19). Skin tags which are symptomatic (pruritus ani, difficulties with anal cleaning post-defaecation) can be excised under local anaesthesia, although in some cases this can also accompany the dilatation.

The author devised a special dilator to be used post-operatively on a long-term basis, as a means to ensure that no return of the pecten band (or other narrowings) was possible. The dilator was large, and there is suspicion that only a minority of patients persisted in its use. There is no information on this point, and the present position would be that use of this dilator is not essential to a successful outcome.

Every patient should be reviewed at two weeks postoperatively, when any persisting symptoms can be treated. In the majority of cases, the patient is discharged, but others may require additional measures, as described earlier. Inadvertent passing of flatus may persist for several months, but should respond within two or three months to sphincter-tightening exercises that can be practised within the home; these cases are reviewed at two months post-operation, when most are discharged.

Complications

In contrast to haemorrhoidectomy, the following complications do not occur: **1)** postoperative bleeding, **2)** urinary retention, **3)** faecal impaction, and **4)** anal stenosis (see Ch. 20: Complications).

Faecal incontinence has been reported. *The author has knowledge of two cases of incontinence but in both cases there was evidence that the dilatation procedure had been wrongly applied*; in one case, too much force was used, leading to sphincter disruption with a keyhole anal deformity; in the other case, the wrong indication was used. Providing anal dilatation is treated with serious respect; carried out for the right indications; and performed with due regard to gentleness and avoidance of sphincter disruption (see Technique), faecal incontinence should not occur.

Finger perforation of the lower rectum has been reported. This is always iatrogenic, being due to forceful pulling with the fully hooked index finger against the rectal wall.

Minor complications (haematomata, small anodermal tears) occur in many cases but require no special treatment other than hot baths and applications of a bland cream (e.g., Nivea); any bruising disperses and the tears heal within a few days.

Despite the simplicity and safety of the dilatation method, it is strongly recommended that informed consent, with full knowledge of all possible complications, should be obtained before carrying out anal dilatation.

Table 7.1. Haemorrhoidectomies Performed in the High Wycombe Hospital Group 1961–1970

Years	Total Number of New Patients	Total Number of haemorrhoidectomies	Number to be expected haemorrhoidectomies on basis of 1961–1964 figures
1961–1964 (average per year)	2,850	54	
1965	3,364	52	63
1966	3,411	38	64
1967	3,955	9	75
1968	3,725	6	71
1969	4,290	6	81
1970	4,381	3	83

Note the abrupt decline of the need for surgical haemorrhoidectomy after 1966, when the method had been accepted by the patients and their family doctors. This was achieved despite rising numbers of patients attending the surgical clinics.

Results

For the elective management of *symptomatic* haemorrhoids that cannot be treated by alternative (office) methods, the results are excellent. Symptoms disappear immediately, and the patient is expected to (and does) return to normal activities the next day. A surgical colleague who was treated by dilatation on a Friday morning under general anaesthesia was able to perform a full operating list on the next day (Saturday). Such dramatic results are not uncommon, but rather the expected outcome. The worse the symptoms, the more gratifying the result (Table 7.1).

Summation

Anal dilatation is a safe, quick and efficient method for treating patients whose haemorrhoids would otherwise require a haemorrhoidectomy. The method can be applied as a day-case procedure under general or caudal anaesthesia. Patients are expected to return to normal activities the

following day. Complications are rare; the most important potential risk is of faecal incontinence, but this can be avoided by careful selection of patients and meticulous gentle technique. Skin tags and mucosal prolapse may require their own treatments post-dilatation.

References and Further Reading

Buchmann P, Babotai I (1984) Why do patients with haemorrhoids benefit from Lord's procedure? pages 166–168 in Coloproctology, 1984. [Editors. J. Cl. Givel and F. Saegesser] Springer-Verlag. Berlin Heidelberg. New York

Hancock BD, Smith K (1975) The internal sphincter and Lord's procedure for haemorrhoids. Brit J Surg 62: 833–36

Hardy KJ, Wheatley IC, Heffernan EB (1975) Anal dilatation and haemorrhoidectomy. A prospective study. Med J Austral 2:88–91

Lord PH (1969) A day case procedure for the cure of third-degree haemorrhoids. Brit J Surg 56:747

Lord PH (1977) Approach to the treatment of ano-rectal disease, with special reference to haemorrhoids. Surg. Ann. 9:195–211

Miles WE (1919) Observations upon internal piles. Surg Gynec Obst 29:496–7

Sun WM, Read NW, Shorthouse AJ (1990) Hypertensive anal cushions as a cause of the high anal pressures in patients with haemorrhoids. Brit J Surg 77:458–62

8 Sclerotherapy for Hemorrhoids

Matthew J. Eckert and Scott R. Steele

Introduction

Hemorrhoidal disease is one of the most common anorectal conditions addressed by proctologists worldwide. While healthcare survey studies estimate the prevalence of this condition amongst adults in the United States to be 4.4%, the actual number of people with hemorrhoidal disease may be significantly higher, as demonstrated in studies utilizing anorectal examination [1, 2]. Though commonly perceived as only a pathological condition, these anal canal fibrovascular cushions function in the fine control of fecal continence. Located in the submucosa, the internal hemorrhoidal venous plexus, in various degrees of distention, contributes up to 20% of resting anal canal pressure [3]. Painless bleeding is the most common presentation of internal hemorrhoids, with itching, hygienic concerns, or a painful mass being less common.

Despite the first description of this disease process centuries ago, the exact pathophysiology of hemorrhoidal disease is still debated today. The most common theory involves chronic elevation of intra-abdominal pressure and frequent straining, resulting in the engorgement of these venous plexi, with subsequent painless bleeding due to tears or ulcerations of the insensate mucosa proximal to the dentate line [4]. Over time, the connective tissue of these chronically engorged submucosal cushions becomes lax, leading to prolapse. Most of the treatment options are then aimed at removing the prolapsed tissue altogether or increasing hemorrhoidal fixation to the anal canal. Yet, with over a dozen therapeutic options described in the current surgical literature, it is not surprising to find a lack of consensus regarding the pathophysiology or ideal treatment.

Sclerotherapy was first described for the treatment of symptomatic internal hemorrhoids by Morgan in 1869 [5]. While numerous sclerosing agents have been utilized in the past, the principle of sclerotherapy for the treatment of bleeding hemorrhoids remains the same. A sclerosant solution is injected into the submucosal tissue at the base of an internal hemorrhoid to create a focus of inflammation. This leads to fibrosis and contraction of the submucosal anal cushion, thus relieving the engorgement of the venous plexus. Ultimately, this causes fixation of the cushion in its normal anatomic position, avoiding prolapse and reducing the size of the cushion to limit future mucosal trauma.

As with its successful use during upper and lower gastrointestinal endoscopy for bleeding [6], sclerotherapy offers several advantages to the practitioner treating hemorrhoids. The technique is relatively simple and easy to learn, with limited procedural time, even for patients requiring multiple injections at one setting. No specialized instrumentation is necessary beyond a side-view anoscope and appropriate needle with syringe. Furthermore, this technique can be safely performed without anesthesia in an office setting.

I. Khubchandani et al. (eds.), *Surgical Treatment of Hemorrhoids*, DOI 10.1007/978-1-84800-314-9_8,
© Springer-Verlag London Limited 2009

Table 8.1 Common Sclerotherapy Agents and Dosage[†]

Agent	Dose
5% Quinine and urea hydrochloride [4]	3–5 ml
1% Sodium tetradecyl sulfate [13]	2–4 ml
5% Phenol in almond/vegetable oil [17]	3–5 ml
23.4% Hypertonic saline [4]	3–5 ml
Sodium morrhuate [16]	3–5 ml
Aluminum potassium sulfate (OC-108) [7]	9–13 ml[†‡]

† Injection dosages provided are the recommended dose per hemorrhoid.
‡ OC-108 is considered an experimental sclerosing agent.

Numerous sclerosing agents are available for use; however, 5% phenol in vegetable or almond oil, 23.4% hypertonic saline, and 5% quinine and urea are among the most popular (Table 8.1). Takano and associates reported favorable results with a novel sclerosing agent containing aluminum potassium sulfate, known as OC-108, when compared with hemorrhoidectomy for Grades III and IV disease [7]. The investigators found that OC-108 was equally effective in resolving prolapse when compared with surgery at the 28-day follow-up; however, the recurrence rate increased to 16% following sclerotherapy versus 2% after surgery, at one year. Regardless of which sclerosing solution is used, the practitioner must be conscious of the differences in dose and inflammatory response unique to each. However, it is the appropriately placed injection that is the key step to successful, safe sclerotherapy for the bleeding internal hemorrhoid.

Indications

Patient selection is an essential component to effective sclerotherapy for symptomatic bleeding internal hemorrhoids. This technique is most appropriate and successful for Grade I and small Grade II internal hemorrhoids, without a mixed internal-external component. Injection sclerotherapy can potentially precipitate acute thrombosis when treating mixed internal-external disease and will certainly result in patient discomfort if used for isolated

external hemorrhoids, and thus is not recommended for external disease. Although the use of sclerotherapy for larger Grade II and III hemorrhoids has been described, both patient satisfaction and successful resolution are less when used in larger hemorrhoidal disease. For that reason, some authors have combined injection sclerotherapy with other treatment modalities, such as banding, in the same treatment session [8]. In such instances where the patient with multi-column symptomatic internal hemorrhoids experiences discomfort with banding, sclerotherapy can be used for the remaining columns to potentially avoid further patient discomfort. This is highlighted by a recent meta-analysis of noninvasive hemorrhoid treatments, in which sclerotherapy was shown to have a lesser incidence of associated pain than hemorrhoidal banding [9].

Prior to injection, a thorough perianal and protocoscopic examination is required. Any evidence of anal fissure, fistula, skin tags, or findings suggestive of inflammatory bowel disease should be considered relative contraindications until further work-up is complete. Active inflammation associated with Crohn's disease or ulcerative colitis should be considered an absolute contraindication to injection sclerotherapy until the inflammatory state is treated and regresses. In this setting, interim management should consist of dietary modification, hydration, and fiber supplementation, in conjunction with appropriate medical management of the acute inflammation.

Other relative contraindications include portal hypertension, active anorectal infection, and immunocompromised states. Yet symptomatic hemorrhoidal bleeding in the HIV/AIDS patient population is a unique circumstance that may be more appropriate for sclerotherapy than other invasive treatment options such as banding or hemorrhoidectomy. In general, due to the poor wound healing and often-seen underlying debilitated physical condition, previous reports have cautioned about the use of hemorrhoidectomy and banding in HIV and AIDS patients after demonstrating a higher incidence of wound and infectious complications [10, 11, 12]. Therefore, injection sclerotherapy may provide a safer alternative for the treatment of symptomatic Grades I and II hemorrhoids in the HIV/AIDS patient;

however, adequate clinical studies to support this are not yet available.

Despite a paucity of literature describing the use of sclerotherapy for symptomatic hemorrhoids in the HIV/AIDS population, Scaglia and associates have reported no complications among a series of twenty-two AIDS patients undergoing injection therapy with 5% phenol or 1% tetradecyl sodium sulfate for bleeding Grade II-IV hemorrhoids [13]. Symptoms improved in fifteen patients after the first injection, while three patients required multiple treatments. Those patients requiring multiple treatments were included in a subgroup of four patients followed for up to four years, demonstrating sustained improvement for 12–18 months with a yearly re-treatment. Given the risks of hemorrhoidectomy in AIDS patients, injection sclerotherapy may ultimately be the preferred treatment option, yet final recommendations await larger studies with longer follow-up.

The treatment of symptomatic internal hemorrhoids in the anticoagulated patient represents another situation for which sclerotherapy may be uniquely suited. Hemorrhoidectomy and banding may result in problematic bleeding or patient distress under these circumstances and discontinuation of anticoagulation medicines may not always be safe or easy to coordinate. Clearly, injection therapy results in less mucosal trauma than these more invasive treatment options, and potentially less bleeding. However, evidence of the efficacy and safety profile of sclerotherapy in the medically anticoagulated patient population remains anecdotal at present [14, 15, 16].

Technique

As with any anorectal procedure a thorough pre-procedural explanation of the steps and expectations is critical to relieve patient anxiety and foster trust between the patient and practitioner. Bowel cleansing preparation is not necessary prior to injection sclerotherapy; however, if possible the patient should be encouraged to have a bowel movement or be given an enema prior to the procedure, thus avoiding passage of firm stools shortly after injection. The patient is typically positioned in the left decubitus or modified prone position with the aid of a proctoscopy examination table. Adequate lighting for visualization of the entire anal canal is essential. Liberal use of topical lubricant is encouraged during placement of a standard side-viewing anoscope, with subsequent careful examination of the entire anal canal.

Prior to initiation of the procedure it is recommended that all necessary instrumentation and supplies be prepared and readily available within reach of the practitioner. Typical supplies consist of a side-viewing anoscope, gauze, lubricant, long cotton swabs, and a sterile Luer Lock-type syringe and appropriate needle. The traditional Gabriel syringe is probably best suited for sclerotherapy, as the three-ring construction allows for injection of viscous oil-based solutions against resistance (Fig. 8.1). Although previous descriptions of this technique recommended the use of a 25-gauge spinal needle, the important principle is to ensure the needle is of adequate length and caliber to facilitate injection [17, 18]. The sclerosing solution should be packaged in sterile individual containers and drawn up into the syringe in sufficient quantity just prior to beginning the procedure.

Careful passage of the side-viewing anoscope will allow each hemorrhoid to fall into the open slot, thus facilitating exposure of the injection site. The dentate line, marking the beginning of the insensate columnar epithelium of the upper anal canal is the key landmark to ensure patient comfort

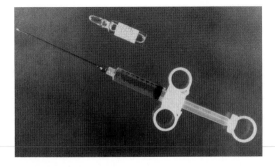

Figure 8.1 Traditional Gabriel needle and syringe. Source: Surgery of the Colon and Rectum, Nicholls RJ and Dazois RR, ed. Elsevier, London 1997:216.

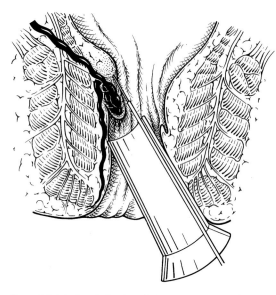

Figure 8.2 Injection of sclerosing solution at appropriate site for internal hemorrhoid. Source: Surgery of the Colon and Rectum, Nicholls RJ and Dazois RR, eds. Elsevier, London 1997:217.

during the injection. The base of the hemorrhoid is identified and the needle is advanced into the sub-mucosal tissue along the vertical plane approximately 1–2 cm (Fig. 8.2). Prior to injection, brief aspiration will determine inadvertent cannulation of a hemorrhoidal vein, for which the needle should be removed and re-inserted. A total of 3–5 ml should be slowly injected into the submucosal tissue at the base of each hemorrhoid. If the injection is too superficial the mucosa will become tense and blanched. The injection should immediately be stopped upon suspicion of superficial placement to avoid mucosal necrosis. The inadvertent transmural injection has few immediate clinical signs to alert the practitioner to the error. Cautious attention to the depth of needle advancement and angle of approach will help to ensure proper injection depth. Particular attention is recommended when injecting anterior wall hemorrhoids, because of the adjacent urologic structures in male patients and the female vagina.

Patients may experience discomfort during the procedure for several reasons. Needle placement too close to the dentate line will result in immediate pain, and is addressed by withdrawing the needle and selecting a more superior injection site. Patients may also feel discomfort during the injection of larger volumes of sclerosing solution, but in general it is a rare occurrence to require more than the standard 3–5 ml per column aliquot. When it does take place, pain is most commonly due to the abrupt tissue expansion or infiltration of the solution toward the dentate line. A slow, consistent injection of appropriate volume will usually help to avoid this discomfort. Accidental injection into a hemorrhoidal vein has been linked to transient epigastric and precordial chest pain, along with an unpleasant taste [19]. Fortunately, this condition is not threatening, and passes quickly with supportive care. Most patients will feel little discomfort beyond that associated with the anoscope. A sense of aching or dull soreness may occur after the procedure, and is addressed with mild oral analgesics.

Injection sclerotherapy may be performed in single or multiple sessions according to patient and practitioner preference. Following an injection, the patient should be counseled about the signs and symptoms of possible treatment side effects. The triad of pelvic pain, fever, and urinary retention associated with pelvic sepsis after anorectal procedures should always be discussed [20]. In addition, patients should be advised to return for evaluation in the event of hematuria, hematospermia, pain or difficulty with urination, or erectile dysfunction. Patients should be encouraged to avoid straining with bowel movements, and should be instructed to begin use of a fiber supplement or another stool bulking agent. A short course of an oral laxative may provide additional help for patients suffering from constipation. We recommend that patients be provided with an educational handout describing the signs and symptoms of potential procedural complications and recommended dietary and stool bulking supplement practices.

Patient follow-up recommendations vary by source and practitioner preference. Our practice is to have patients return for re-examination three to six weeks after injection, or earlier if symptoms persist. However, mandatory follow-up in the asymptomatic patient is not required. There is no evidence to support single versus multiple session injection, and this is practitioner-dependent [21]. In the event of recurrent bleeding following a symptom-free interval, patients are encouraged to return early in their symptom course while the hemorrhoid is still amenable to re-injection as dictated by grade of prolapse.

Results

The efficacy of sclerotherapy in resolving symptomatic internal hemorrhoids has been evaluated in numerous small-scale clinical trials and several retrospective reviews. Mann et al. reported a 75% rate of resolution or improvement in symptomatic bleeding among one hundred patients with Grade I hemorrhoids who underwent sclerotherapy with 5% phenol oil and who were followed for one month [22]. Khoury and colleagues prospectively randomized 120 patients with Grade I and II disease to single versus multiple injections, with nearly 90% reporting resolution or improvement in symptoms one year after injection and no difference with regard to the number of treatment sessions required [21]. However, in a smaller trial of 49 patients with symptomatic bleeding hemorrhoids randomized to either a bulk laxative or a bulk laxative with concomitant injection sclerotherapy, there was no difference in bleeding recurrence after six months, suggesting that sclerotherapy may be no better than dietary and medical management alone [23].

Numerous investigators have found the benefits of injection therapy to be short-lived, with no clear advantage when compared to banding or photocoagulation, in complication profile or patient preference. Kanellos et al. prospectively evaluated 238 patients with Grades I and II disease that underwent sclerotherapy. At three year follow-up, only 20% of Grade I patients and 8.7% of Grade II patients were symptom free. However, 42% of patients with Grade I and 64% of patients with Grade II hemorrhoids reported worsening of symptoms, with the remainder being unchanged or improved [24].

A meta-analysis by Johanson and Rimm evaluated five studies including patients with Grades I and II disease who underwent banding, injection sclerotherapy, or infrared photocoagulation [25].

Twelve months after treatment, the banding group had a trend towards a higher rate of symptom resolution when compared to sclerotherapy [60 of 163 patients (37%) versus 44 of 175 patients (25%), respectively, $p = 0.07$], with no difference in pain or bleeding complications. When stratified by disease severity, symptoms associated with Grade II hemorrhoids were significantly improved after banding when compared to sclerotherapy. Pooled results of Grade I and II disease demonstrated that patients having undergone banding were significantly less likely to require additional treatment when compared to sclerotherapy [14 of 163 patients (9%) versus 39 of 171 patients (23%), respectively, $p = 0.009$].

McRae and associates conducted a large meta-analysis of 18 individual trials including over 1,600 patients encompassing all grades of disease and operative and nonoperative treatment in 1995 [9]. The authors concluded that banding is the preferred initial treatment modality for Grades I to III hemorrhoids, based upon statistically significant symptomatic improvement and equivocal complication rates when comparing banding with sclerotherapy or infrared photocoagulation (Table 8.2). Patients receiving sclerotherapy were more likely to require additional treatment sessions when compared to banding, but were less likely to experience procedural-related pain. The authors analyzed two studies comparing sclerotherapy to infrared photocoagulation, finding no difference in response rates or number of treatment sessions required.

Finally, given the variety of treatment modalities available it is not surprising that combined treatment options for Grades I and II disease have also been explored. Chew and colleagues randomly surveyed 2,400 patients who underwent combined sclerotherapy and banding for Grade I or II hemorrhoids at the same time [8]. At a mean follow-up of 6.5 years, 58% reported no residual symptoms, while an additional 32% reported symptomatic improvement. Recurrence, defined as requiring re-treatment after a period of 12 months from the last treatment, occurred in 16% of patients, with 7.7% of patients eventually requiring hemorrhoidectomy. The authors concluded that there was no difference in symptomatic improvement rates after combined treatment when compared to studies

Table 8.2 Summary of Clinical Trials Evaluating Nonoperative Treatment of Internal Hemorrhoids and Including Sclerotherapy

	# of Patients			Follow-up (mos)	No Response to Treatment					Further Treatment Required				
	IS	RBL	IRC		IS	RBL	IRC	OR	p	IS	RBL	IRC	OR	p
Gartell [26]	109	105		33	35	11		0.25	0.001	27	7		0.25	0.001
Cheng [27]	30	30		12	6	2		0.11	0.09					
Greca [28]	33	28		12	10	10		1.3	0.20	4	2		1.2	0.75
Sim [16]	24	22		12	6	6		1.1	0.86	5	5		1.1	0.88
Overall	196	185			57	29		0.43	0.005	36	14		0.45	0.03
Ambrose [29]	42		52	12	11		9	0.59	0.30	6		12	1.8	0.22
Walker [15]	35		38	48	4		1	0.21	0.14	1		2	1.9	0.61
Overall	77		90		15		10	0.48	0.10	7		14	1.8	0.27

IS, injection sclerotherapy; RBL, rubber band ligation; IRC, infrared photocoagulation; OR, odds ratio; p, p-value
Source: Adapted from McRae HM, McLeod RS [9].

utilizing only banding, and the incidence of hemorrhoidectomy was similar when compared to the known literature.

Kanellos and associates prospectively randomized 255 patients to one of three treatment arms—banding with sclerotherapy, banding alone, or sclerotherapy alone. Four years after treatment 46% of patients treated with the combined approach were symptom free, compared to only 8% of the sclerotherapy alone group ($p < 0.001$); however, there was no difference compared to the 36% rate of symptom resolution in the banding alone group ($p = 0.217$) [30]. Thus, at this time there does not appear to be a significant advantage to a combined treatment utilizing sclerotherapy when compared to the available individual treatments.

Complications

The technique of injection sclerotherapy is a safe and simple procedure, with few relatively uncommon complications. The selection of appropriate patients and accurate injection will help to eliminate most procedural-related complications and ensure satisfactory results. However, no invasive procedure is without risk. The most frequent complication associated with injection sclerotherapy is minor patient discomfort that may be addressed with stool softeners and/or mild oral analgesics. As mentioned, inadvertent injection into a hemorrhoidal vein may be associated with transient precordial or epigastric pain without detrimental long-term effects. Bleeding from injection site(s) is usually self-limited, but may be addressed with direct pressure, topical epinephrine, or banding if persistent and significant. Caution should be exercised when planning to inject patients using anticoagulation or antiplatelet medications, although from personal anecdotal experience, this has proven successful. Erroneous injection of larger Grades III and IV hemorrhoids with subsequent prolapse may result in acute thrombosis with significant patient discomfort, requiring surgical intervention.

All anorectal procedures bear the potential risk of local and systemic infection. Localized abscess formation in the anorectal wall or adjacent prostate is a rare but potential complication, and distant hepatic abscesses have been reported in a single patient following injection [31]. Adami and colleagues demonstrated an eight percent incidence of bacteremia without systemic complications following proctoscopy and injection sclerotherapy [32]. These findings prompted Kaider-Person et al. to recommend antibiotic prophylaxis prior to injection in patients with predisposing cardiac valvular disease or immunodeficiency [4]. Pelvic sepsis, necrotizing soft tissue infection, and anorectal necrosis following sclerotherapy are extremely rare but reported events [33, 34].

Other rare complications associated with injection sclerotherapy have resulted from erroneous placement or from the systemic effects of the sclerosant solution itself. A single case report of respiratory failure with the development of adult respiratory distress syndrome following sclerotherapy with 5% phenol oil has been documented [35]. Following a short duration of ventilatory support the patient recovered without long-term detrimental effects. Systemic absorption of phenol has also been linked to transient chemical hepatitis after injection therapy [36]. While the associated jaundice resolves relatively quickly, liver function tests may require several months to return to normal, and patients should be counseled appropriately.

Given the proximity of the male prostate and periprostatic nerve bundles to the anterior anorectal wall, various genitourinary complications following sclerotherapy have been reported. Urinary retention is the most common symptom following intraprostatic injection, which typically occurs with injection of anterior wall hemorrhoids [19]. Emphasizing this, a survey of British surgeons utilizing injection therapy reported a 31% complication rate, of which the majority was urological and associated with anterior hemorrhoidal injection [37]. Other reported urological complications include hematospermia and hematuria, dysuria, prostatitis, epididymo-orchitis, and erectile dysfunction [38, 39].

Conclusion

Injection sclerotherapy is a safe and simple treatment modality, and most effective for the small, symptomatic internal hemorrhoid. While most studies suggest that the long-term relief of symptomatic bleeding is likely best achieved by hemorrhoidal banding, injection sclerotherapy remains a viable adjunct treatment, and provides a useful tool for the surgeon treating hemorrhoidal disease. This procedure may prove to be especially useful in the patient taking anticoagulation

medication or in the HIV patient population, although further data is needed. Finally, this technique may also be safely combined with other less invasive treatment modalities, but appropriate patient selection and technique are essential to ensure positive results.

References

1. Johanson JF, Sonnenberg A. The prevalence of hemorrhoids and chronic constipation. An epidemiologic study. Gastroenterology 1990;98:380–86.
2. Haas PA, Haas GP, Schmaltz S, Fox TA Jr. The prevalence of hemorrhoids. Dis Colon Rectum 1983;26:435–39.
3. Lestar B, Penninckx F, Kerremans R. The composition of anal basal pressure. An in vivo and in vitro study in man. Int J Colorectal Dis 1989;4:118–22.
4. Kaider-Person O, Person B, Wexner S. Hemorrhoidal disease: a comprehensive review. J Am Coll Surg 2007;204: 102–117.
5. Morgan J. Varicose state of saphenous haemorrhoids treated successfully by the injection of tincture of persulphate of iron. Medical Press and Circular 1869;29–30.
6. Ponsky JL, Mellinger JD, Simon IB. Endoscopic retrograde haemorrhoidal sclerotherapy using 23.4% saline: a preliminary report. Gastrointest Endosc 1991;37:155–58.
7. Takano M, Iwadare J, Ohba H, et al. Sclerosing therapy of internal hemorrhoids with a novel sclerosing agent. Comparison with ligation and excision. Int J Colorectal Dis 2006;21:44–51.
8. Chew SS, Marshall L, Kalish L et al. Short-term and long-term results of combined sclerotherapy and rubber band ligation of hemorrhoids and mucosal prolapse. Dis Colon Rectum 2003;46:1232–237.
9. MacRae HM, McLeod RS. Comparison of hemorrhoidal treatment modalities. Dis Colon Rectum 1995;38:687–94.
10. Wexner SD, Smithy WB, Misom JW et al. The surgical management of anorectal diseases in AIDS and pre-AIDS patients. Dis Colon Rectum 1986;29:719–23.
11. Afavi A, Gottesman L, Dailey T. Anorectal surgery in the HIV+ patient: update. Dis Colon Rectum 1991;34: 299–304.
12. Morandi E, Merlini D, Salvaggio A et al. Prospective study of healing time after hemorrhoidectomy. Influence of HIV infection, Acquired Immunodeficiency Syndrome, and anal wound infection. Dis Colon Rectum 1999; 42:1140–144.
13. Scaglia M, Delaini GG, Destefano I et al. Injection treatment of haemorrhoids in patients with acquired immunodeficiency syndrome. Dis Colon Rectum 2001;44:401–04.
14. The ASCARS Textbook of Colon and Rectal Surgery. Wolff BG, Fleshman JW, Beck DE, Pemberton JH, Wexner DE, eds. Springer, New York 2007:164–65.
15. Walker AJ, Leicester RJ, Nicholls RJ, Mann CV. A prospective study of infrared coagulation, injection and rubber band ligation in the treatment of haemorrhoids. Int J Colorectal Dis 1990;5:113–16.

16. Sim AJ, Muries JA, Mackenzie I. Three year follow-up on the treatment of first and second degree hemorrhoids by sclerosant injection or rubber band ligation. Surg Gynecol Obstet 1983;157:534–36.

17. Beck DE. Hemorrhoids. In: Beck DE, ed. Handbook of colorectal surgery, 2nd ed. Marcel Dekker, New York 1997:325–44.

18. Mazier WP. Hemorrhoids. In: Mazier WP, Luchtefeld MA, Levien DH, Senagore AJ, eds. Surgery of the colon, rectum and anus. W.B. Saunders, Philadelphia 1995:229–54.

19. Mann CV. Sclerotherapy. In: Mann CV, editor. Surgical treatment of haemorrhoids, 1st ed. Springer, London 2002:57–64.

20. Quevedo-Bonilla G, Farkas AM, Abearian H et al. Septic complications of hemorrhoidal banding. Arch Surg 1988;123:650–51.

21. Khoury GA, Lake SP, Lewis MC et al. A randomized trial to compare single with multiple phenol injection treatment for haemorrhoids. Br J Surg 1985;72:741–42.

22. Mann CV, Motson R, Clifton M. The immediate response to injection therapy for first-degree haemorrhoids. J Royal Soc Med 1988;81:146–48.

23. Senapati A, Nicholls RJ. A randomized trial to compare the results of injection sclerotherapy with a bulk laxative alone in the treatment of bleeding internal haemorrhoids. Int J Colorectal Dis 1988;3:124–26.

24. Kanellos I, Goulimaris I, Vkalis I et al. Long-term evaluation of sclerotherapy for haemorrhoids: a prospective study. Int J Surg Investig 2000;2:295–98.

25. Johanson JF, Rimm A. Optimal nonsurgical treatment of hemorrhoids: a comparative analysis of infrared coagulation, rubber band ligation, and injection sclerotherapy. Am J Gastroenterol 1992;87:1601–606.

26. Gartell PC, Sheridan RJ, McGinn FP. Out-patient treatment of haemorrhoids: a randomized clinical trial to compare rubber band ligation with phenol injection. Br J Surg 1985;72:478–79.

27. Cheng FC, Shum DW, Ong GB. The treatment of second degree hemorrhoids by injection, rubber band ligation, maximal anal dilatation and hemorrhoidectomy, a prospective clinical trial. Aust N Z J Surg 1981;51:458–62.

28. Greca F, Hares MM, Nevah E et al. A randomized trial to compare rubber band ligation with phenol injection for treatment of haemorrhoids. Br J Surg 1981;68:250–52.

29. Ambrose NS, Hares M, Alexander-Williams I et al. Prospective randomized comparison of photocoagulation and rubber band ligation in treatment of haemorrhoids. BMJ 1983;286:1387–389.

30. Kanellos I, Goulimaris I, Christofordis E et al. A comparison of the simultaneous application of sclerotherapy and rubber band ligation, with sclerotherapy and rubber band ligation applied separately, for the treatment of haemorrhoids: a prospective randomized trial. Colorectal Dis 2003;5:133–38.

31. Murray-Lyon IM, Kirkham JS. Hepatic abscesses complicating injection sclerotherapy of haemorrhoids. Euro J Gastroenterol Hepatol 2001;13:971–72.

32. Adami B, Eckhardt V, Suermann R et al. Bacteremia after proctoscopy and hemorrhoidal injection sclerotherapy. Dis Colon Rectum 1981;24:373–74.

33. Guy RJ, Seow-Choen F. Septic complications after treatment of haemorrhoids. Br J Surg 2003;90:147–56.

34. Elram R, Wasserberg N. Anorectal necrosis induced by injection sclerotherapy for hemorrhoids. Int J Colorectal Dis 2006 Jun 21; [Epub ahead of print].

35. Rashid M, Murtaza B, Gondal Z, Mehmood A, Shah S et al. Injection sclerotherapy for haemorrhoids causing adult respiratory distress syndrome. J Coll Physicians Surg Pak 2006;16:373–75.

36. Suppiah A, Perry E. Jaundice as a presentation of phenol induced hepatotoxicity following injection sclerotherapy for haemorrhoids. Surgeon 2005;3:43–44.

37. Al-Ghnaniem R, Leather AJ, Rennie JA. Survey of methods of treatment of haemorrhoids and complications on injection sclerotherapy. Ann R Coll Surg Engl 2001;83:325–28.

38. Wright AD. Complications of rectal injuries. Proc R Soc Med 1950;43:263–66.

39. Bullock N. Impotence after sclerotherapy of haemorrhoids: case reports. BMJ 1997;314:419–20.

9 Rubber Band Ligation

Jose Alfredo dos Reis Neto and José Alfredo dos Reis Junior

Hemorrhoids begin as localized cushions of submucosal vascular tissue. These cushions are present at birth and represent a normal anatomical feature of the anal canal. The cushions are located in the submucosa of the anal canal underlying the transitional zone that joins the squamous epithelium of the anoderm to the rectal columnar epithelium [1, 9, 10, 11].

The cushions are supplied by the superior hemorrhoidal artery that gives off branches anteriorly and posteriorly on the right side and a single branch on the left, usually lateral. This anatomical position of the hemorrhoidal artery's branches corresponds to the more common location of the hemorrhoidal cushions and subsequent piles. The presence of arteriovenous anastomoses within the cushions has been demonstrated by studies of oxygen saturation of the hemorrhoidal blood as well as by injection techniques [9]. The function of the submucosal vascular tissue is to cushion the anal canal during defecation [8]. It is also believed that it contributes to continence when engorged [8].

As the cushions are a normal anatomical element of the anal canal, the existence of hemorrhoids is determined by the occurrence of distinct pathological changes (Fig. 9.1).

The sequence of obstruction of the venous outflow produces distention of the cushions and the degeneration of the collagen and elastic tissue stroma, leading to downward displacement of the hemorrhoidal cushions and the production of vascular congestion. At defecation this displacement is repeated and enlarged, increasing the grade of elastic tissue degeneration. After repeated episodes the cushions slip through the anal canal and there may occur some grade of superficial erosion of the anal mucosa that overlies the cushion [1, 9].

Prolapse and bleeding are the most common symptoms referred to hemorrhoidal disease and become progressively worse through the years. Rectal bleeding with defecation is the most common manifestation. The bleeding occurs as a bright red spot or streak on the toilet tissue or as blood dripping into the toilet bowl. Cushion prolapse may be sensed as a mass protruding through the anus during defecation that reduces spontaneously at the beginning. Chronic prolapse may result in persistent mucoid discharge, causing perianal pruritus and dermatitis. Pain is not a common symptom of hemorrhoidal disease unless there is any complication, such as acute thrombosis or fissure [11].

Constipation, diarrhea, pregnancy, and sedentary lifestyle increase the severity of symptoms [11]. Hemorrhoidal disease has been stratified into four grades [1]:

1. Grade I—cushions are enlarged, congested, but do not prolapse;
2. Grade II—cushions are enlarged, congested, prolapse with defecation, but reduce spontaneously;
3. Grade III—cushions are enlarged, congested, prolapse consistently with defecation, and must be reduced digitally;
4. Grade IV—cushions are permanently prolapsed and cannot be reduced.

I. Khubchandani et al. (eds.), *Surgical Treatment of Hemorrhoids*, DOI 10.1007/978-1-84800-314-9_9,

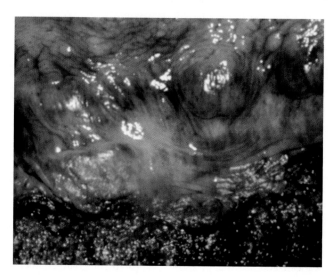

Figure 9.1 Hemorrhoidal cushions

However, with the recognition that the cushions are a normal anatomic element of the anal canal, a more clinically useful classification system is based on symptoms: either the presence or absence of bleeding, prolapse, and pain.

The choice of hemorrhoidal treatment should be based on the nature and severity of symptoms, which are related to the nature and severity of the cushions' displacement [1, 14, 21, 22, 23].

Minimally symptomatic disease can often be managed clinically: dietary fiber supplements when necessary, physical activities, warm sitz baths, avoiding the use of toilet paper, and topical preparations. It is extremely important to exclude a more serious condition as the cause of the bleeding, particularly when the patient has anemia, weight loss, diarrhea, or has a family history of polyps or cancer [1]. Nonsurgical therapies are being used with increasing frequency, especially for internal hemorrhoids with mild symptoms [1, 5, 7, 13, 14, 15, 18]. Among the nonsurgical procedures, rubber band ligature is the one most widely used [1, 2, 3, 4, 7, 17, 18, 20, 23, 28, 29]. The goal of a rubber band ligature is to promote fibrosis of the submucosa with subsequent fixation of the anal epithelium to the underlying sphincter, impeding the downward displacement of the hemorrhoidal cushions [1, 20, 21, 22, 23, 28, 29].

Indications

Banding ligature is only suitable for internal hemorrhoids.

Contraindications

A general examination should be performed to exclude conditions such as portal hypertension requiring specific treatment [12]. Rigid proctosigmoidoscopy must be carried out before the banding to exclude rectal cancer or IBD. Colonoscopy must be performed in patients with a familial high risk of cancer or polyps. Banding should not be performed in the presence of an anal fissure (acute or chronic), abscess, or fistula.

Preparation

No special preparation is necessary. A normal defecation on the day before the procedure or even on the morning of the procedure is the best preparation. Constipation should be corrected before the procedure.

Anesthesia

If properly performed, the banding is painless. However, to facilitate the banding, it is recommended to inject 0.5–1.0 ml of lidocaine at the submucosa of the anal canal with a fine needle on the area where the banding is to be applied. This maneuver facilitates the grasping or the suction of the mucosa.

Position of the Patient

The Sims (left lateral) position with the pelvis raised on a sandbag is the best position for the procedure. The rubber banding can also be realized in the knee-elbow or jackknife positions. The lithotomy position should be avoided.

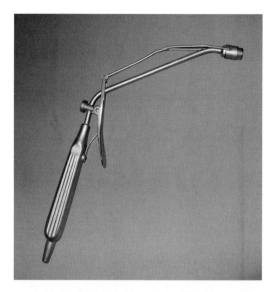

Figure 9.3 Suction rubber band device

Instruments

There are two methods of banding: one by grasping the submucosa (traction) and one by suctioning it (Figs. 9.2 and 9.3). The banding instrument consists of a double drum carrying elastic bands. This double drum is mounted on a long shaft, at the base of which is a trigger mechanism which can release the elastic bands as required. The small elastic rings are loaded by a conical device that enables the bands to be slipped over from the loader onto the drum. The bands are 1/16 inch in diameter when unexpanded and 1.0 cm when loaded onto the drum. When using the grasping device, it is necessary to have a special pair of grasping forceps, which are passed

through the hollow core of the drum, to grasp each pile in turn. With this method the surgeon needs one assistant to hold the anoscope. The suction device is adapted to a suction pump and the pile is drawn downward by sucking the mucosa of the anal canal; with this method the surgeon can hold the anoscope with one hand and use the other one to release the bands.

Illumination

A normal anoscope, 1.6 cm in diameter and 6 cm long, is suitable for banding. These are available in two types, one with a distally placed (close to the mucosa) source of illumination, and the other with the source of light placed at its proximal end. The former provides excellent illumination, which, however, frequently becomes dimmed by blood or excretions. A double spotlight, with converging illumination, could be used for excellent illumination.

Procedure

The pile must be banded 1 cm above the pectinate line. The pile is grasped or suctioned at its base;

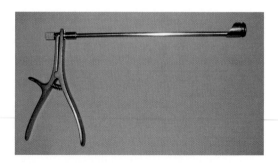

Figure 9.2 Rubber band device using traction by grasping the mucosa

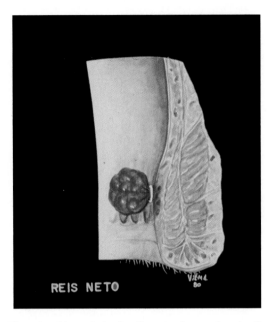

Figure 9.4 Scheme of a banding, illustrating the area where the pile must be banded

grasping or suctioning the pile by its middle point can produce laceration and bleeding (Fig. 9.4). The injection of 0.5–1 ml of lidocaine at the base of the pile with a fine needle facilitates the banding and avoids the discomfort originating from the suction or grasping. It is preferable to treat all the hemorrhoids (2–4 piles) in one single session [19, 20]. Sequential single banding can be performed, but at least 21 days should elapse between the sessions [17].

Some Important Technical Points

1. Sprinkle lidocaine spray in the anal area and perform a gentle anal dilatation with lidocaine gel before the introduction of the anoscope; this tends to diminish the discomfort of the anoscope penetration.
2. Banding the pectinate line will produce severe pain and discomfort, with the formation of an ulcer.
3. Avoid putting the bands very close to one another when banding all the piles in one single session, because this can produce bleeding when the rubber ring is eliminated.

4. Use a gentle traction or suction of the mucosa, not using force to traction the pile.
5. Injection of 0.5–1.0 ml at the base of the pile before the banding eases the grasping or the suction and diminishes any immediate aching discomfort.
6. A little enema of 10 ml of lidocaine (2% without adrenaline) after finishing all banding procedures avoids immediate postoperative tenesmus and discomfort.

Results

All data expressed are derived from:

- Prospective randomized trial on conservative therapy for internal hemorrhoids [13, 20].
- International inquiry of 318 specialists [1]

Immediate

A great majority of the patients (82%) report no symptoms while banding and 14% felt some kind of discomfort. No treatment was interrupted for pain or discomfort.

Late

In the first week after treatment, 27% of the patients had shown some level of tenesmus and discomfort. Pain was observed in 14% of the patients, 78% were treated by oral analgesics (dipirona or ibuprofen) or anti-inflammatory drugs (nimesulide, diclofenate, or similar); 22% needed some kind of parenteral analgesic. After two weeks, 14% of the patients still had some kind of discomfort and tenesmus. Tenesmus was treated by small enemas of 2% lidocaine (10 ml without adrenaline) every 12 or 24 hours, according to the intensity of the symptoms.

Complications

Some small bleeding on defecation was observed in 13% of the patients, between the sixth and tenth postoperative days. Severe bleeding was observed in 0.1% of the patients, 90% of them needing hospitalization. Anoscope reexamination showed necrosis at the site of the banding and ulceration. None needed to be reoperated. Perianal edema occurred in 2% of the patients; all were treated by warm sitz baths. Perianal hematoma occurred in 2% of the patients. Fatal sepsis caused by multiple organisms has been reported after the banding. No apparent risk factors for this have been identified, but salvage is only possible by immediate examination of all the patients reporting severe pain or fever after the treatment [27]. Emergent surgical debridement is the surgical treatment if a necrotizing infection is found on examination.

Recurrence

A prospective randomized trial revealed that 93% of the patients with prolapse and bleeding treated by rubber band ligature were still asymptomatic one and two years after treatment [20]. A ten-year follow-up registered a 10.5% recurrence rate [1, 20].

High Macro Rubber Band

During the last decade, the idea of intervening higher in the anal canal to impede the downward displacement of the hemorrhoidal cushions at their origin has become more and more accepted. The strategy of removing a segment of the anal canal to eliminate the zone with degeneration of the collagen and elastic tissue stroma and suspending the lower anal canal has been shown to be effective for hemorrhoidal disease Grades II and III. Known as anopexy and performed with a mechanical device, this procedure establishes a new line of hemorrhoidal disease treatment [6, 7, 16, 26].

Based on the same principle, a new technique of ligature was developed with two purposes [21, 22, 24, 25]:

1. to promote better fibrosis and fixation by banding a bigger volume of tissue; and
2. to perform this fixation at the origin of the hemorrhoidal cushion displacement, preventing the cushion from slipping through the anal canal.

Indications

High macro banding ligature is suitable for internal hemorrhoids Grades II and III.

Contraindications

These are the same as for the conventional banding technique.

Preparation

No special preparation is necessary.

Anesthesia

If properly performed the high macro banding is painless. However, to facilitate the banding, it is helpful to inject 1.5 ml of lidocaine at the submucosa of the anal canal with a fine needle. This injection must be performed higher in the anal canal, 4–5 cm above the pectinate line, according to the location of internal piles. If the patient has more than one pile, two or more areas could be injected. This maneuver facilitates the suction of the mucosa.

Position of the Patient

The Sims (left lateral) position with the pelvis raised on a sandbag is the best position for the procedure.

Instruments

There is only one method of high macro banding: by suction. The banding instrument for high macro ligature consists of a double drum 3 cm in length and 1.5 cm in diameter (Fig. 9.5a–b). This double drum is mounted on a long shaft, at the base of which is a trigger mechanism which can release the elastic bands as required. The small elastic rings are loaded by a conical device that enables the bands to be slipped over from the loader onto the drum. The bands are 2 mm in diameter when unexpanded and 1.5 cm when loaded onto the drum. The suction device is adapted to a suction pump and the pile is drawn downward by sucking the mucosa of the anal

canal; with this method the surgeon can hold the anoscope with one hand and use the other hand to release the bands. It is helpful to use a longer and wider anoscope to obtain a better view of the anal canal, which will facilitate injecting the submucosa higher in the anal canal and inserting the rubber band device.

Procedure

The pile must be banded higher in the anal canal (4–5 cm above the pectinate line). The mucosa, previously injected, is gently suctioned at the same

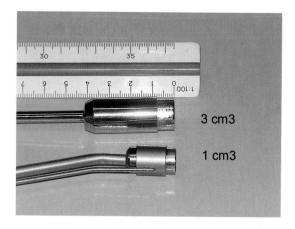

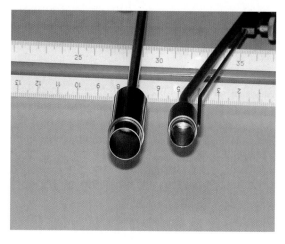

Figure 9.5a–b Comparison between the normal rubber band instrument and the macro one

time that the rubber band device is slowly moved downward, parallel to the anoscope, for just a small distance. This maneuver facilitates the suction of a great volume of mucosa and avoids the discomfort originating from the suction. It is preferable to treat all the hemorrhoids in one single session (to a maximum of three). When using the macro rubber band, it is preferable to band the existent piles at different levels, to avoid stricture of the anal canal. One pile can be banded four centimeters higher and the others at five or six cm (Figs. 9.6 and 9.7). Sequential single banding can be performed, but at least 30 days should elapse between sessions.

Some Important Technical Points

1. Sprinkle lidocaine spray in the anal area and perform a gentle anal dilatation with lidocaine gel, before the introduction of the anoscope; this maneuver tends to diminish the discomfort of the anoscope penetration.
2. Begin the procedure by the injection of 1.5–2.0 ml of lidocaine with a fine needle (use the dental surgeon syringe) at the mucosa higher in the anal canal, utilizing a normal anoscope.

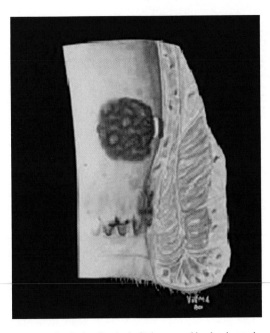

Figure 9.6 Site for banding in the high macro rubber band procedure

3. Avoid putting the macro bands very close to one another and at the same level when banding all the piles in one single session, since this can produce anal canal stricture.
4. Use a gentle suction of the mucosa, not using force or traction on the pile.
5. A little enema of 10 ml of lidocaine (2% without adrenaline) after finishing the macro banding procedure avoids immediate postoperative tenesmus and discomfort.

Results and Complications

All data expressed are derived from personal experience [21, 22, 24, 25].

We analyzed the results obtained in 805 patients with internal hemorrhoids Grades II and III. There was no distinction as to age, gender, or race. The analysis was retrospective without any comparison with conventional banding. The period of evaluation extended from one to seven years.

Immediate

The following immediate complications were observed: edema in 1.6%, tenesmus in 0.6%, pain (need for parenteral analgesia) 1.6%, minor bleeding in 5.5%, profuse bleeding in 0.6%, and urinary retention in 0.1% of the patients. None of the patients needed hospitalization for the observed complications.

Late

The great majority ($n = 96$, 1%) of the patients were free of symptoms five years after the high macro banding. Recurrence of the symptoms occurred in 3–9% of the patients, all of them treated by a new macro banding.

Conclusions

The analysis of the observed results shows a small incidence of minor complications, with a high index of symptomatic relief. The high macro banding technique represents an alternative method for

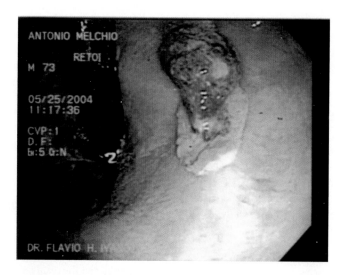

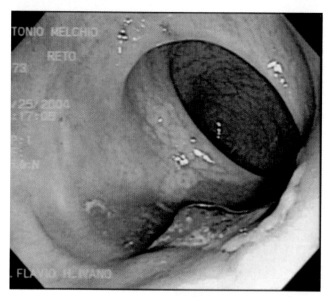

Figure 9.7 High macro rubber banding 7 days after the procedure

the treatment of internal hemorrhoids Grades II and III, with good results at low cost. The two main differences between the method described and conventional rubber banding are:

1. The level of the banding—the macro rubber band ligature is performed 4–5 cm above the pectinate line.
2. Volume—the volume of banded mucosa is 3–4 times greater than with the usual banding technique.

References

1. Abcarian H, Alexander-Williams J, Christiansen J, Johanson J, Killingback M, Nelson RL, Reis Neto JA. Benign anorectal disease: definition, characterization and analysis of treatment. Am J Gastroenterol 1994;89(8):s182.
2. Barron J. Office ligation treatment of hemorrhoids. Dis Colon Rectum 1963;6:109–12.
3. Baumgartner R. Treatment of internal hemorrhoids by way of elastic ligature. Schweiz Med Wochenschr 1970; 100:1249.

4. Blaisdell PC. Office ligation of internal hemorrhoids: a 10-year report with simplified technique. Am J Proct 1966; 17:25–28.

5. Dennison AR, Wherry DC, Morris DL. Hemorrhoids: non-operative management. Surg Clin N Am 1988;68:1401–09.

6. Ganio E, Lus AR, Trompetto M, Clerico G et al. Stapled haemorrhoidectomy. In: Reis Neto JA, ed. New trends in coloproctology. Ed. Revinter, Brasil, 2000:207–18.

7. Gathright JB, Araghizadeh F. Closed hemorrhoidectomy. In: Reis Neto JA, ed. New trends in coloproctology. Ed. Revinter, Brasil, 2000:175–90.

8. Gibbons CP, Bannister JJ, Towbridge EA, Read NW. The role of anal cushions in maintaining continence. Lancet 1986;1:886.

9. Haas PA, Fox TA, Haas GH. The pathogenesis of hemorrhoids. Dis Colon Rectum 1984;27:442–50.

10. Hosking SW, Johnson AG, Smart HL, Trigger D. Anorectal varices, hemorrhoids, and portal hypertension. Lancet 1989;1:349–52.

11. Hyams L, Philpot J. An epidemiological investigation of hemorrhoids. Am J Proctol 1970;21:177–93.

12. Jacobs DM, Bubrick MP, Onstad GR, Hitchcock CR. The relationship of hemorrhoids to portal hypertension. Dis Colon Rectum 1980;23:567–69.

13. Johanson JF, Riomm A. Optimal nonsurgical therapy of hemorrhoids: meta-analysis of the comparative efficacy of infrared coagulation, injection sclerotherapy and rubber band ligation. Am J Gastroenterol 1992;87:1601–06.

14. Jones IT, Fazio VW. Anorectal diseases commonly encountered in clinical practice. In: Kirsner JB, Shorter RG, eds. Diseases of the colon, rectum, and anal canal. Williams and Wilkins, Baltimore 1988:688–89.

15. Khubchandani IT, Rosen L, Russel RW et al. Are we ready for ambulatory anorectal surgery? 88th Annual Convention, American Society of Colon and Rectal Surgeons, Toronto, 1989.

16. Longo A. Treatment of hemorrhoids disease by reduction of mucosa and hemorrhoidal prolapse with circular suturing device; a new procedure. 6th World Congress of Endoscopy Surgery, Rome, 1998:777.

17. Mann CV. Barron band ligation of haemorrhoids. In: Rob C, Smith R, Todd IP, eds. Operative surgery. Colon, rectum and anus, 3rd ed. Butterworths, 1977:315–18.

18. Newstead GL. Ambulatory treatment of benign anal diseases. In: Reis Neto JA, ed. New trends in coloproctology. Ed. Revinter, Brasil, 2000:197–206.

19. Poon GP, Chu KW, Lan WY et al. Conventional vs triple rubber band ligation for hemorrhoids: a prospective randomized trial. Dis Colon Rectum 1986;29:836–40.

20. Reis Neto JA, Quilici FA, Cordeiro F, Reis JA Jr. Ambulatory treatment of haemorrhoids: a prospective random trial. Coloproctology 1992 Nov–Dec;14(6):342–47.

21. Reis Neto JA, Quilici FA, Cordeiro F, Reis JA Jr, Kagohara O, Simões Neto J, Sugahara RD. Macroligadura alta: um novo conceito no tratamento ambulatorial das hemorróidas. Rev Bras Coloproctologia, 2003 Jan–Mar; 23(1):9–14.

22. Reis Neto JA, Quilici FA, Cordeiro F, Reis JA Jr, Kagohara O, Simões Neto J. Macroligadura alta: um nuevo concepto en el tratamiento del prolapso hemorroidário. In: Moreno Gonzalez E, ed. Actualización en Cirugía del Aparato Digestivo 2005:XI:315–19.

23. Reis Neto JA, Quilici FA, Cordeiro F, Reis JA Jr. Open versus semi-open hemorrhoidectomy: a random Trial. Int Surg 1992;77:84–89.

24. Reis Neto JA, Reis JA Jr, Kagohara O, Simões Neto J. High macro rubber band ligature: a new concept in the treatment of haemorrhoids. Proktologia 2003;4(3):236–37.

25. Reis Neto JA, Reis JA Jr, Kagohara O, Simões Neto J, Amarillo H. Macroligadura alta: un nuevo concepto en el tratamiento de hemorroides. Rev Mex Coloproctologia 2007;13(1):15–20.

26. Ruiz-Healy F, Diaz AM. Semiclosed hemorrhoidectomy. In: Reis Neto JA, ed. New trends in coloproctology. Ed. Revinter, Brasil, 2000:191–96.

27. Russel TR, Donohue JH. Hemorrhoidal banding: a warning. Dis Colon Rectum 1985;28:291–93.

28. Smith LE. Hemorrhoids; a review of current techniques and management. Surg Clin North Am 1987;16:79–91.

29. Soullard J. Ligadura elástica. In: Lentini J. Temas de Coloproctologia, Ed. Fontalba, tomo I, 1982:cap IV-2:167–68.

10 Treatment of Hemorrhoids by Infrared Thermocoagulation

Philip F. Caushaj, Soni Chousleb, and Elias Chousleb

Introduction

The ideal therapy for hemorrhoids in early stages has always been debated. Some methods are effective but are associated with more pain, while some are less painful but also less effective. Thermocoagulation methods have been used for a long time, including direct current probe, bipolar diathermy, cryoablation, and infrared coagulation, with variable success rates.

Infrared coagulation was introduced in the 1970s by Nath. This method returns the anal cushions to their normal size and position, offering a more anatomical cure, which is preferable to the destruction of tissue that other thermal methods produce. The infrared coagulating system works by infrared radiation and not by any electrical current. Mechanical pressure and radiation have to be applied simultaneously. Pulses of infrared radiation are applied to the hemorrhoidal packages using a handheld applicator, causing shrinkage of the hemorrhoids and causing the mucosa to become fixed to the underlying tissue.

Most of the instruments consist of a power unit and a manual applicator that has interchangeable light conductors and a trigger to activate the device. A standard projector bulb focused on a quartz light guide by a gold-plated reflector generates the infrared energy. A 10-mm quartz light conductor is generally used for the treatment of hemorrhoids.

Infrared coagulation operates at a temperature just above 100° C. Tissue coagulation with radiation is based on the denaturalization of proteins.

After 1 second of exposure a hissing noise can be heard, which indicates that intracellular fluid has reached the boiling point. The superficial cellular fluid is at a temperature of more than 100° C. Longer exposure times lead to desiccation and subsequent carbonization, which is useful to arrest acute bleeding hemorrhoids [1].

This technique can be controlled and reproduced simply by measuring the time of exposure, obtaining the same depth of necrosis, and avoiding the area of the surrounding tissue. This allows high power density to be generated at a single point. In order to prevent adhesion, the tip of the light conductor is coated with a fluorocarbon copolymer that is transparent to the infrared light. Hemostasis is achieved with a minimum energy dose and coagulation intervals are shorter. The reliability of this technique lies in the simplicity of operation and that the exact depth of necrosis can be preset using a timer adjustment. This is in contrast with electrocoagulation, which is dependent on the electrolyte concentration of the cells, and the depth of necrosis cannot be reproduced in a standardized way.

Advantages

1. The infrared coagulator does not cause electromagnetic interference, making it safe to use in patients with pacemakers.

I. Khubchandani et al. (eds.), *Surgical Treatment of Hemorrhoids*, DOI 10.1007/978-1-84800-314-9_10, © Springer-Verlag London Limited 2009

2. Coagulation time can be achieved in only 1–3 seconds.
3. There is no tissue adhesion.
4. The precise depth of necrosis can be determined.
5. The coagulator is suitable for use in active bleeding.
6. There is safe low voltage.
7. It is safe for use during pregnancy.
8. No inactive electrodes have to be placed.

The aim is to obliterate the hemorrhoids by scar tissue shrinkage. The pulse length determines the depth of necrosis, but there is a limit of 3 mm penetration. If applied for a very long time or for repeated applications in the same session, the tissue carbonizes, which is useful only if the patient presents with active bleeding at the moment of the intervention.

Disadvantages

1. Recurrence of the hemorrhoids.
2. Several sessions needed to accomplish cure.
3. Soiling.
4. Proctitis.

Indications

1. Hemorrhoids, first- and second-degree.
2. Acutely bleeding hemorrhoids.

Several prospective studies have shown the efficacy of treatment using thermocoagulation, comparing it to the use of rubber band ligation and sclerotherapy. In general, this procedure is well tolerated by patients, because the pain is minimal and it has been shown to have the same effectivness for the treatment of Grade I internal hemorrhoids. The procedure can be done at the office with a minimal complication rate and at low cost. Patients may return to their activities sooner. On the other hand, studies have shown the need for repeated sessions to treat hemorrhoids in a satisfactory fashion.

The few randomized clinical trials that are available concluded that infrared coagulation (IRC) and rubber band ligation (RBL) are equally effective in the treatment of hemorrhoids, and that IRC should be advocated as the first line of therapy for first-degree hemorrhoids that do not respond to conservative measures [2, 3, 4, 6].

Technique

The patient is positioned in lateral decubitus. The hemorrhoids are first located with a digital rectal exam, then (optionally) a proctoscope is used to visualize them and the infrared coagulator is inserted through an anoscope. There is no need to use local anesthesia. The tip of the instrument is positioned just above the hemorrhoid, and the infrared lamp is activated to produce coagulation either in a diamond shape or in a rainbow shape to ensure the coagulation of the entire hemorrhoidal package. A second coagulation is then performed, rotating the instrument 90 degrees. Since the tip is coated with flurocarbon polymer, the mucosal surface does not attach to the instrument and it can be lifted easily from the site of treatment without tearing the tissue.

The irradiated area will appear gray at the end of the procedure. After one week has gone by, an in-drawn spot with capillarization that appears red can be visualized. In two weeks, scar tissue is present in the area, and after four weeks normal mucosa appears in the site of treatment.

Conclusions

Several treatment options are available for the treatment of hemorrhoids, including nonsurgical management with dietary modifications;

procedures that can be perfomed in the physician's office, like rubber band ligation, cryoablation, infrared thermocoagulation, etc.; and the different surgical treatment modalities. However, there is still not a definitive consensus on what the gold standard for treatment should be. Different treatment series have had good results with some techniques, but other series have not been able to reproduce the same results. Part of the problem also is the degree of hemorrhoids.

Treatment may vary diversely, with varying results. The only common agreement in most of the series is that thermocoagulation reduces the pain during and after the intervention, which makes it more acceptable to the patients; but it needs recurrent treatment sessions to achieve a cure.

References

1. Leicester RJ. Treatment for hemorrhoids by infrared thermocoagulation.
2. Poen AC et al. Randomized controlled trial of rubber band ligation versus infrared coagulation in the treatment of internal hemorrhoids. Eur J Gastroenterol Hepatol 2000;12(5).
3. Dimitroulopoulus D et al. Prospective, randomized, controlled, observer-blinded trial of combined infrared photocoagulation and micronized purified flavinoid fraction vs. each alone for the treatment of hemorrhoidal disease. Clin Ther 2005 Jun;2(6).
4. Charua L et al. La fotocoagulacion por rayos infrarrojos en el tratamiento de la enfermedad hemorroidaria. Rev Gastroenterol Mex 1998;63(3):13–134.
5. Charua L et al. Manejo alternativo no quirurgico de la enfermedad hemorroidaria. Rev Gastroenterol Mex 2005;70(3).
6. Linares E et al. Eficacia del tratamiento hemorroidal mediante la ligadura con bandas elasticas y la fotocoagulacion infrarroja. Rev Esp Enf Dig 2001;93(4).

11 Open Hemorrhoidectomy

Yasuko Maeda and Robin K. S. Phillips

Open hemorrhoidectomy is the technique originally described by Milligan in 1937 and normally referred to as the Milligan-Morgan operation [1]. Essentially it is a low ligation with excision of the hemorrhoids.

Selection of Cases

This is an operation *par excellence* for treating patients with significant external components. Patients with so-called first-degree hemorrhoids, who have anal canal bleeding (essentially, blood on wiping and occasionally dripping into the pan) only really need an appropriate examination and reassurance that nothing more sinister is present. Those with prolapse represent a broad group of patients. Occasionally, internal hemorrhoidal prolapse can be massive yet without a significant external component. Office treatments can be ineffectual when truly gross internal hemorrhoids are encountered, and here again open hemorrhoidectomy has a role.

Patients with strangulated or thrombosed piles may also be treated by open hemorrhoidectomy, particularly when the thrombosed/strangulated areas are discrete and it is easy to determine what should be removed and what left behind. In more gross cases where such distinction is hard if not impossible, traditionalists are likely to adopt a nonoperative approach, although

there are many surgeons who will still choose some form of surgical intervention.

Patients with either a fissure or a fistula which in its own right warrants an operation can have an open hemorrhoidectomy performed at the same time.

Some patients with an apparent external component and bleeding have these symptoms as a response to anal digitation for obstructive defecation; open hemorrhoidectomy will not aid their bowel evacuation difficulty.

Traditionally surgeons confronted by patients with Crohn's disease are strongly advised to avoid surgery, particularly where inflammation in the anorectum is marked. On occasion, the Crohn's disease may seem incidental to the hemorrhoidal problem. Great caution and reluctance to consider an operation should still be the "default setting," but on occasion so-called hemorrhoids in Crohn's patients can make a patient's life such a misery that the potentially greater risks of delayed healing or even precipitation of proctectomy will not deter the patient from consenting to their removal. In such special circumstances, although it is wise to keep clear and accurate records of the advice and warnings given, it is reasonable to respect the patient's wishes and acquiesce to open hemorrhoidectomy.

Seeding of colorectal cancer cells into hemorrhoidectomy wounds has been described on a number of occasions. The more universal routine use of flexible sigmoidoscopy over rigid proctoscopy should substantially lessen the risk.

I. Khubchandani et al. (eds.), *Surgical Treatment of Hemorrhoids*, DOI 10.1007/978-1-84800-314-9_11,
© Springer-Verlag London Limited 2009

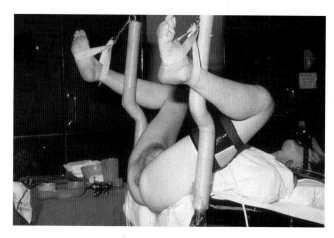

Figure 11.1 The "extended" lithotomy position for anal surgery: good for the operating surgeon, but harder for the assistant to teach from.

Preparation

Little formal preparation is required besides an anesthetic check. Patients on warfarin can undergo open hemorrhoidectomy, although they need conversion to heparin first, then a short gap without anticoagulation for surgery, followed by re-heparinization for a period until the risk of secondary hemorrhage has reduced significantly and warfarin can be commenced again.

Bowel preparation is unnecessary. Stool softeners, given for a few days before surgery so that the first bowel movement after surgery is soft, have been shown to reduce postoperative pain [2] and seem sensible. Whereas some surgeons like to use a disposable enema before operation, others find the occasional pools of residual liquid more troublesome than more solid material and prefer to avoid an enema. Perioperative antibiotics have not been tested in this setting but seem eminently reasonable.

Position

Traditionally the lithotomy position has been used. If it is used, it is important to obtain a good lithotomy position which does not have the patient at a right angle at the hips and perched on the edge of the operating table, but rather has the buttocks thrust forward off the end of the operating table with an acute angle at the hips (Fig. 11.1). In this more extended lithotomy position, the anus is directly in front of the surgeon and the hemorrhoids are made more prominent and thus easier to operate on because of the increased abdominal pressure resulting from the slight flexion of the knees towards the chest. The lithotomy position remains an extremely good and comfortable position for the first surgeon, but it is more difficult for an assistant than when the patient is prone. When conducting an inexperienced surgeon through an anal operation, the prone position may be preferred.

Anesthesia

The operation is usually performed under general anesthesia supplemented by local infiltration of local anesthetic and often a pudendal nerve block, but regional anesthesia can be used.

Technique

The patient is placed appropriately on the operating table, prepped, and draped. In the lithotomy position a small table/tray placed between the surgeon and the buttocks is highly convenient.

The operation needs to be planned according to the findings under anesthesia. An appropriate anal retractor (the authors prefer the Eisenhammer) permits a good view of hemorrhoids under direct vision. Examine each hemorrhoidal mass and then concentrate on the skin bridges. Are they "clean" or are there secondary hemorrhoids that may need to be dealt with as well? If clean and if the hemorrhoids are in the classic positions with no other complicating factors, then, having alerted the anesthetist, infiltration of the surgical site can be commenced with 1 in 200,000 adrenaline. Local anesthetic can either be added to this solution or given separately at the end of the procedure.

It makes most sense to infiltrate the skin bridges, as the cut edges of these will be the sites of any bleeding. In addition, the external component should be infiltrated. The surgeon should pause and use moist gauze to massage the infiltrated areas to permit time for the adrenaline to act and to disperse the solution that otherwise can make identification of the planes more difficult.

Small artery forceps are then placed on the external component at the three main sites. Traction on these prolapses the internal components, which are likewise grasped in small artery forceps (Fig. 11.2). Commencing with the 3 o'clock hemorrhoid, the relevant two artery forceps are grasped in the palm of the left hand and the index finger extended anally to define the triangle of exposure, and using curved Mayo scissors the skin is incised (Fig. 11.3). The external component is dissected off the underlying superficial external anal sphincter (Fig. 11.4). More cephalad dissection separates the

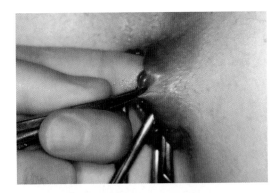

Figure 11.3 The first cut is made with Mayo scissors.

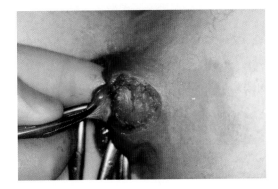

Figure 11.4 The operation proceeds, clearing the hemorrhoidal tissue from the underlying external anal sphincter.

internal component from the underlying internal anal sphincter, continually narrowing down the pedicle (Fig. 11.5). At this stage the surgeon may choose to transfix and ligate the pedicle (the

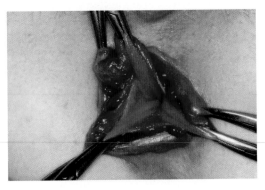

Figure 11.2 The initial triangle of exposure.

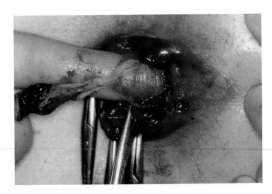

Figure 11.5 The internal sphincter is separated from the pile pedicle.

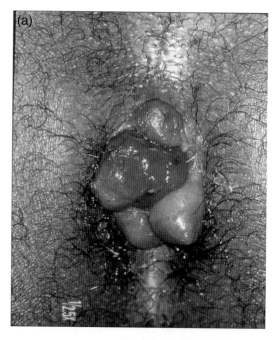 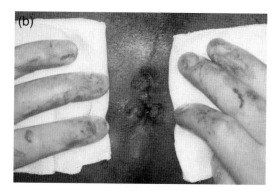

Figure 11.6a and b Before and after images in a different case: "If it looks like a clover, your troubles are over; if it looks like a dahlia, it's a failure."

classical operation) or using electrocautery, simply diathermy it.

The operation then proceeds via the 11 o'clock and 7 o'clock hemorrhoids, and hemostasis is checked. The skin bridges with the Milligan-Morgan technique are much slimmer than in closed hemorrhoidectomy.

Anal dressings are a potent cause of anal discomfort and retention of urine after surgery and should be avoided if at all possible. Figure 11.6a and b represent before and after images from a different case illustrating the open wound that will usually take 6–8 weeks to heal completely. There is an old adage: "If it looks like a clover your troubles are over. If it looks like a dahlia it's a failure."

a) "Filleting" (Fig. 11.7). If there are only a limited number of residual hemorrhoids, they can be teased out from beneath the edges of the skin bridges. This should not result in the skin bridges being separated from their attachment to the wall of the anal canal (in which case it would be better to use technique "b" below).

b) Skin bridge division and resuture. If there are gross residual hemorrhoids beneath one of the skin bridges, then that skin bridge may be divided in its upper half, reflected out of the anus, the hemorrhoidal tissue cleaned from the back of it (Fig. 11.8), redundant mucosa excised, and then the flap resutured into place (Fig. 11.9). This is safe to do in one bridge when the others are satisfactory, but probably should otherwise be avoided.

Residual Hemorrhoids

The surgeon may choose to leave these and if necessary return on another occasion. Alternatively, they can be handled by one of two alternative methods as follows:

Postoperative Care

The patient may be discharged home after recovery from the anesthesia. The patient should go home with regular analgesics along with rescue

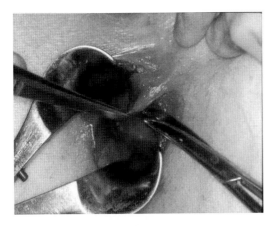

Figure 11.7 'Filletting' secondary hemorrhoids from under a skin bridge.

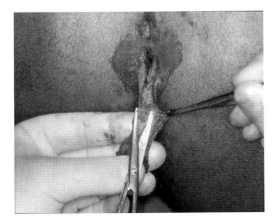

Figure 11.8 The posterior skin bridge has been divided above the dentate line, flipped out of the anus, and residual hemorrhoids are being removed with scissors.

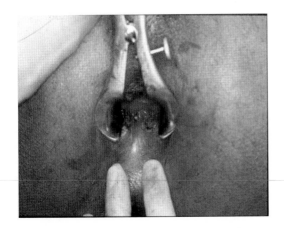

Figure 11.9 The reconstituted 6 o'clock skin bridge.

pain killers. Nonsteroidal anti-inflammatory drugs are effective enough to control the pain sufficiently. To keep the stool softer, laxatives should also be prescribed and used regularly until a regular and pain-free bowel habit has been established. Oral metronidazole may help to manage the postoperative pain [3], as may some form of chemical sphincterotomy (e.g., using 0.2% diltiazem gel). The knowledge that there will be an early review (but after the first week, when patients may be quite querulous) gives much needed psychological support should there be an early pain increase.

Complications

Complications occur despite meticulous surgical technique, and patients need to be warned carefully before being discharged from the hospital. Increased pain after surgery, particularly between days 3 and 5; acute retention of urine; secondary bleeding; stenosis; and incontinence are some of the known complications after the procedure. Printed information would be helpful for patients to take home, and reassurance should be given that certain minor adverse events are frequently encountered and not to be unduly worried about. Arranging a follow-up at early stage (within two weeks) will give extra reassurance to the patients and prevent anxious phone calls in the first week when discomfort is greatest.

Occasionally a "fissure" can develop at the site of one of the healing wounds. Usually it is not of the "pain/constipation" type and simply reflects delayed wound healing. Frequently an application of silver nitrate will be all that is needed; very rarely curettage may be necessary. Treatment is not the same as for a standard fissure, and chemical or surgical sphincterotomy are not usually called for.

Rarely, removal of too much skin results in stenosis. Early on this may manifest by a persistent fissure; every time it tries to heal, it is split open again by the passage of stool. If detected in the first couple of months after surgery, then examination under anesthetic with Hagar's dilatation followed by self-dilatation twice daily for two months will usually resolve the problem. However, if the diagnosis is made late, then no amount of dilatation will solve the problem, and some sort of plastic surgical procedure, excising scar tissue from the anal canal and relining it with supple skin (such as by house advancement) will be necessary to fix the problem.

References

1. Milligan ETC, Morgan CN, Jones LE, Officer R. Surgical anatomy of the anal canal and the operative treatment of haemorrhoids. Lancet 1937;2:1119.
2. London NJM, Bramley PD, Windle R. Effect of four days of preoperative lactulose on posthaemorrhoidectomy pain: results of placebo controlled trial. Br Med J 1987; 295:363–64.
3. Carapeti EA, Kamm MA, McDonald PJ, Phillips RKS. Double-blind randomised controlled trial of effect of metronidazole on pain after day-case haemorrhoidectomy. Lancet 1998;351:169–72.

12 Closed Hemorrhoidectomy (Khubchandani Technique)

Indru T. Khubchandani

Closed hemorrhoidectomy is associated with the technique first described by Ferguson and Heaton in 1959 [1]. I have chosen to give it a different eponym, inasmuch as the technique has been modified considerably from the one first described.

The procedure performed by us is in a prone jackknife position and not in a left lateral Sim's. The anesthesia used is largely local (0.5% lidocaine with 1:200,000 epinephrine), as described by us in 1972 [2]. The suture material used is fine; we have elected to use 5.0 polyglycolic acid for many years, on account of its appropriate tensile strength, and the dissolution in about ten to twelve days when the wounds are generally healed, if closed without tension. We apply a simple over-and-over *apposition* closure, not hemostatic with tension, and leave a dead space without incorporating the underlying sphincter musculature.

Indications

With the newly available techniques for nonsurgical hemorrhoidectomy, surgical hemorrhoidectomy is being practiced much less frequently. However, for fourth-degree hemorrhoids and some third-degree hemorrhoids, a well-performed hemorrhoidectomy, with removal of the pathology and correction of the associated conditions, still remains the procedure of choice. A technique of closed hemorrhoidectomy with primary closure of the incisions and local anesthesia is described.

Preoperative Preparation

Unless the history indicates otherwise, no preoperative testing is needed, especially if the patient has had some other procedures performed in the past. An ECG is performed in the elderly only when there is a history of cardiac problems. A chest radiograph is not necessary. Unless the patient has previously been on anticoagulants, the preoperative coagulation work-up is not necessary. The patient should be approved for anesthesia preoperatively during the preadmission testing. The patient should fast after midnight the day before surgery and report to the Ambulatory Surgical unit on the morning of surgery, after having self-administered a disposable phosphosoda enema. An intravenous line is established with a 250 ml solution of 0.5% normal saline in 5% dextrose. The patient is delivered to the Operating Room by foot. A wheelchair is used if the patient has had sedation in the holding room.

I. Khubchandani et al. (eds.), *Surgical Treatment of Hemorrhoids*, DOI 10.1007/978-1-84800-314-9_12,
© Springer-Verlag London Limited 2009

Position and Anesthesia

A prone jackknife position is used and the buttocks are retracted with adhesive tape on both sides (Fig. 12.1). The hips are flexed, and both arms are extended. The patient is sedated with Propofol® (Zeneca) and/or Midazolam® (Roche). The local anesthesia used is 0.5% lidocaine with 1:200,000 epinephrine. About 15 ml of this solution is used per procedure. A subcutaneous, circumferential infiltration is performed with a no. 30 needle using approximately 5 ml of this solution. Another 8 ml are then deposited in the submucous plane, 2 ml in each of the four quadrants, with a finger or a pediatric Hill-Ferguson retractor in the anal canal (Fig. 12.2). If the solution is inadvertently deposited in the plane outside of the sphincter muscle, no ill effects are encountered. The anesthetic effect is instantaneous and complete with adequate relaxation of the sphincter.

Procedure

A medium sized Hill-Ferguson retractor is inserted, and the anal canal is inspected. A plan is outlined for the extent of the required

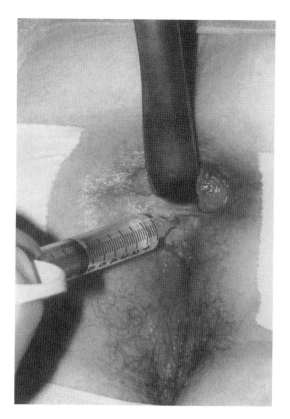

Fig. 12.2 Infiltration of local anesthetic solution in the submucosal plane.

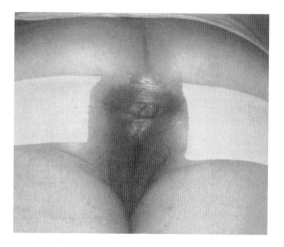

Fig. 12.1 Patient in prone (jack-knife) position with buttocks retracted with adhesive tape.

dissection. As a rule, three classic primary hemorrhoidal complexes (i.e., left lateral, right posterior, and right anterior quadrants) are excised. However, the author chooses to remove the larger, seemingly symptomatic complex or complexes only. Care is taken to avoid making excisions in the anterior and posterior midline, where an unhealed wound may result. A knife is used to make a radical elliptical incision, encompassing the primary hemorrhoidal complex, starting at the point proximal to the dentate line and extending well beyond the anal verge. Using scissors, the skin is lifted from the underlying external sphincter, and the mucosa is freed from the internal sphincter cephalad, proximal to the dentate line. With local anesthesia, the tissue planes are remarkably easily demarcated, and the anatomic definitions are perfect. Due to vascular constriction, the blood loss is minimal, often requiring only a few 4 × 4 sponges for the entire procedure. A suction device is not necessary.

The proximal point is reached when the attachment of the muscle of Treitz (longitudinal fiber complex) is seen to anchor the internal sphincter to the mucosa. Using scissors, this mucosal suspensory ligament is divided: the salmon-colored proximal part of the internal sphincter is dissected free, and the hemorrhoidal complex is excised (Fig. 12.3). This is the so-called "pedicle" described in the literature, and it does not bleed. The use of sphincterotomy in the base of the wound has been abandoned. In a prospective randomized study, internal sphincterotomy did not relieve pain and caused deficit incontinence [3]. The wound is closed primarily with one continuous, simple over-and-over suture of 5-0 polyglycolic acid, beginning at the apex, the most proximal point of the excised tissue, and ending at the external verge, where no attempt is made to leave any open area for drainage (Fig. 12.4). Reinforcing sutures are not used.

The suture should not be pulled tight. It is intended to approximate the tissue, rather than act as a hemostatic constriction. Contrary to the traditional surgical axiom, no attempt is made to eliminate the potentially contaminated deep space. The underlying sphincter muscle, therefore, is not incorporated into the suture. No drainage tubes or hemostatic packs are inserted, and no compression dressing is considered necessary. Only an external Tefla® dressing may be applied. A completed three-column hemorrhoidectomy is shown in (Fig. 12.5).

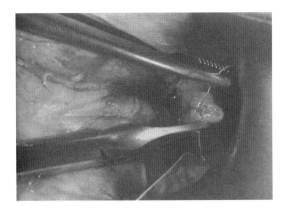

Fig. 12.4 Closure of the wound, commencing at the proximal cut edge of the "pedicle".

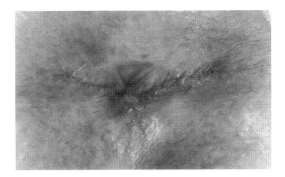

Fig. 12.5 Complete closure of the wounds.

Postoperative Management

The patients return directly to the Ambulatory Suite, either via wheelchair or on a stretcher. They are given a snack and a drink soon afterwards, and if necessary, an oral analgesic. Patients are discharged one-half to one hour after surgery with appropriate instructions.

The follow-up regimen consists of sitz baths (patients are given a disposable sitz bath to be placed over the commode with connections for plumbing), and patients are advised to take an oral analgesic Dulcolax® on the evening of surgery to promote a bowel movement. In addition, patients are advised to take a bulk supplement, such as psyllium seed, to facilitate bowel activity. An appointment is scheduled 10 days postoperatively, when the sutures will

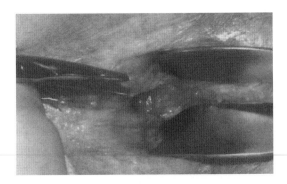

Fig. 12.3 Dissection of hemorrhoidal mass, well proximal to the dentate line.

be absorbed. The next visit is scheduled for three weeks later (if necessary), when the wounds are completely healed.

Results

Table 12.1 lists the complications in a series of 3,274 cases. The low incidence of urinary retention (3.7%) is explained by the limited use of intravenous hydration during the procedure [1]. There is a low incidence of infection and abscess formation (0.16%). Postoperative pain is always difficult to evaluate. However, most patients do not finish a 30-tablet prescription for analgesic medication (oxycodone). Postoperative follow-up (one to seven years) of 441 patients who underwent closed hemorrhoidectomy, patient satisfaction was 92.6% [4].

Table 12.1 Complications of closed hemorrhoidectomy in 3,274 cases

Complications	Number (%)
Bleeding:	
Requiring packing	16 (0.49)
Requiring reoperation	0 (0)
Abscess formation:	
Opened in office	4 (0.12)
Requiring reoperation	2 (0.06)
Suture line dehiscence:	
One-quarter only	163 (4.97)
Circumferential	2 (0.06)
Urinary retention	121 (3.70)
Excessive edema requiring reoperation	199 (6.08)

Discussion

Closed hemorrhoidectomy with local anesthesia is the preferred choice for surgical management of hemorrhoidal disease in the United States. A questionnaire sent by Wolfe et al. to members of the American Society of Colon and Rectal Surgeons revealed that 65.6% of surgeons who performed a closed hemorrhoidectomy used local anesthesia [5]. This author prefers the closed hemorrhoidectomy technique because it affords faster healing (*per primam*), less pain, and fewer complications. The procedure can be performed in an ambulatory setting, requiring about a two-hour stay at the hospital. Resumption of full activity, particularly in the motivated patient, occurs in about one to two weeks.

References

1. Ferguson, DJ, Heaton JR. Closed hemorrhoidectomy. Dis Colon Rectum 1959;2:176–79.
2. Khubchandani IT, Trimpi HD, Sheets JA. Closed hemorrhoidectomy with local anesthesia. Surg Gynecol Obstet 1972;135:955–57.
3. Khubchandani IT. Internal sphincterotomy with hemorrhoidectomy does not relieve pain: a prospective, randomized study. Dis Colon Rectum 2002;45:1452–57.
4. McConnell JC, Khubchandani IT. Long-term follow-up of closed hemorrhoidectomy. Dis Colon Rectum 1983; 26:797.
5. Wolf JS, Munoz JJ, Rosin JD. Survey of hemorrhoidectomy practices: open versus closed techniques. Dis Colon Rectum 1979;22:536–38.

13 The Surgical Treatment of Hemorrhoids by Submucosal Hemorrhoidectomy (Parks Method)

Neil James Mortensen and Michael Warner

Introduction

Parks developed the submucosal hemorrhoidectomy operation in the 1950s and published his results and details of the technique in 1956 [5]. The operation is designed to treat the hemorrhoids while causing as little pain as possible and avoiding the complications of anal and rectal stenoses. Parks believed that the widely practiced Milligan-Morgan excision ligation technique caused excessive pain because the hemorrhoidal "pedicle" was ligated at a level where sensate anoderm is present. Furthermore, Parks disagreed with the anatomical basis on which the Milligan-Morgan operation had been devised. Historical procedures, such as the Salmon technique, which involved high ligation in the rectum, resulted in too much rectal mucosa being removed, thus leading to stenosis. Parks's technique combines high ligation in the insensate rectum with a mucosal sparing technique that aims to avoid stenosis.

Indications

In Parks's original series of fifty patients, 85% suffered from "prolapse." His description of the technique gives the impression that most of the patients had second- or third-degree hemorrhoids with little in the way of an external component. At this time there are numerous options for treating prolapsing internal hemorrhoids without resorting to hemorrhoidectomy. Many surgeons would try an outpatient-based treatment such as rubber band ligation. Where this fails, some surgeons recommend stapled hemorrhoidopexy. Our practice is to offer hemorrhoidectomy to patients who have irreducibly prolapsed (fourth-degree) hemorrhoids, patients with large symptomatic external hemorrhoids, and some of those who have failed outpatient-based treatments.

Preoperative Preparation

Ensuring the patient has soft stools by prescribing a stool softener prior to surgery probably makes the first defecation after surgery less painful. The patient is admitted on the day of surgery with no special preparation required. A short time prior to surgery a phosphate enema is administered, as this makes for a clear operating field. Thromboembolic prophylaxis is not required unless the patient has a specific risk factor. Most commonly a general anesthetic without a muscle relaxant is chosen. Spinal anesthesia is also acceptable. We do not use prophylactic antibiotics routinely for anal surgery. The patient is placed in the lithotomy position, as this is simple and adequate.

I. Khubchandani et al. (eds.), *Surgical Treatment of Hemorrhoids*, DOI 10.1007/978-1-84800-314-9_13,
© Springer-Verlag London Limited 2009

Prone-jackknife gives good exposure, particularly for the assistant, and is useful for training; however, it is time consuming and has risks for the patient. The patient is prepped with an aqueous prep and draped in standard fashion.

Technique

A Parks anal retractor is inserted. The right posterior hemorrhoid is treated first. A point just caudal to the dentate line at the hemorrhoid is grasped with a hemostat. Parks used 30–40 ml of a solution containing adrenaline 1 part to 400,000 saline. This is injected submucosally to display the anatomy. Our practice is to use dilute bupivacaine with adrenaline solution, as this aids postoperative analgesia.

Scissors are used to excise a small diamond of anal epithelium around the hemostat. When there are large external hemorrhoids or tags, as is usually the case in our practice, this diamond is converted into an ellipse. This excises the redundant skin of the external hemorrhoid and therefore avoids leaving skin tags. The incision is then continued cranially for 2.5 cm. Some authors have recommended making a Y-shaped incision rather than a straight incision, which they feel makes the submucosal dissection easier (Fig. 13.1).

The edges of the mucosa on each side of this incision are grasped with two further hemostats and dissection occurs submucosally to expose the hemorrhoidal tissue to be removed and create two mucosal flaps. Mostly the dentate line is tethered to the underlying internal sphincter by fibrous tissue. This fibrous tissue was named the mucosal ligament by Parks, and it must be divided to allow the dissection to occur. Next, by pulling on the hemostat, grasping the diamond of skin axially, the hemorrhoidal plexus is dissected off the underlying internal sphincter muscle. This dissection is continued into the rectum where the resulting broad base of tissue is suture ligated and divided (Figs. 13.2 & 13.3).

The mucosal flaps are then allowed to flop back into position. In Parks's original description sutures were not used in the mucosa unless the operation was for prolapsing hemorrhoids, in which case Parks felt it was important to suture the mucosal flaps

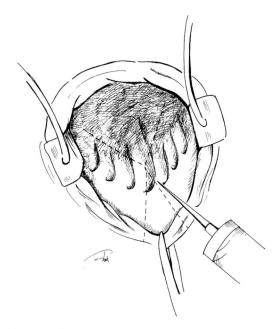

Figure 13.1 Lines of incision and local injection; note the Y-shaped incision on the internal hemorrhoid favored by modern advocates of the Parks Technique.

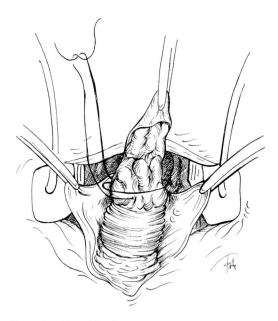

Figure 13.2 Mucosal flaps have been created and hemorrhoid has been dissected free of internal sphincter in readiness for pedicle ligation.

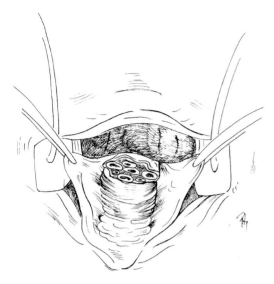

Figure 13.3 Hemorrhoid excised after ligation.

down to the muscle to reconstitute the "mucosal ligament." Most contemporary descriptions of the technique describe suturing the mucosal flaps loosely together and to the underlying sphincter (Fig. 13.4). The same procedure is carried out on the other hemorrhoids. In cases of secondary hemorrhoids, these can either be removed by continuing the submucosal dissection from one of the incisions or, if large, a further incision can be made. It is not our

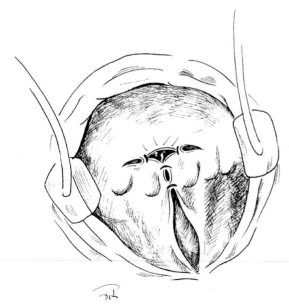

Figure 13.4 Loose closure of the mucosal flaps.

practice to perform internal sphincterotomy at the time of hemorrhoidectomy. We do not use any intra-anal dressing. We insert both a metronidazole suppository and a NSAID suppository at completion of the operation.

Postoperative Management

The patient is recovered in the day case unit's ward and closely observed for possible early complications. Urinary retention is common and should be treated by catheterization early to avoid bladder distension injury; overnight admission is arranged in this situation. Postoperative bleeding is unusual. Providing that patients have passed urine, are comfortable, and have an appropriate social situation, they are allowed home the same day.

The patient commences on a combination of a fiber supplement such as Fybogel and an osmotic laxative such as lactulose. Analgesia with NSAIDs and a relatively nonconstipating opioid such as tramadol are usually sufficient at home. Occasionally a stronger oral opioid such as morphine elixir is required.

The importance of taking laxatives and the need to avoid constipation is stressed. Patients are counselled to expect a further week or two of pain and advised to reduce their laxative if their bowel actions are getting too loose. We advise our patients to have a daily bath to keep their anus and wounds clean and to use a simple dry dressing only. We review our patients in the outpatient clinic at six weeks. They are checked to see if they have ongoing pain, unhealed wounds, or evidence of anal stenosis. Providing patients and clinicians are happy, no further arrangements are made to see them again.

Evidence for Parks's Submucosal Hemorrhoidectomy

Roe published a randomized clinical trial comparing submucosal versus excision ligation hemorrhoidectomy in 1987 [6]. This trial randomized

43 patients to each arm. The submucosal arm had the operation exactly as described by Parks. The excision ligation arm had the Milligan-Morgan operation, although the surgeons did make sure they ligated the pedicle well above the dentate line. As well as checking for postoperative pain, they performed pre- and postoperative manometry and anal sensation measurements. There were no differences in pain in the first five days or at six weeks. Manometry did not demonstrate any differences. Anal sensation, as measured by an electrical catheter, was better in the submucosal group, but this did not translate into clinically apparent improved function at six weeks. They concluded that the submucosal technique was not inferior to excision ligation, but there was no evidence to warrant adopting the technique for all patients.

Hosch performed another randomized clinical trial comparing submucosal hemorrhoidectomy to the Milligan-Morgan technique [1]. He randomized 34 patients, with 17 in each group. The two groups were similar. Parks's operation took longer (42 minutes vs. 33.6 minutes). Length of stay was longer for Milligan-Morgan (4.6 days vs. 3.2 days). Milligan-Morgan patients were off work for longer (20.2 days vs. 12.2 days). Hosch concluded that the Parks operation was superior to the Milligan-Morgan. Other evidence comes only from various case series. These show low rates of severe pain, low complication rates, and low rates of the wounds breaking down [3, 4, 7].

Conclusions

Parks's submucosal hemorrhoidectomy has repeatedly been shown to be safe and is associated with low rates of complication and recurrence. It has also been shown that it takes longer and is more difficult to learn. It has not been clearly shown to be superior to any other technique. It is for these reasons that we and many others no longer practice this technique. The theoretical arguments behind the Parks operation are, however, compelling.

Parks's patients mostly had only second- or third-degree hemorrhoids, and his operation was really designed to treat predominantly internal hemorrhoids. As discussed, pure internal hemorrhoids are commonly amenable to less invasive outpatient-based treatments. When the external component needs to be addressed, such as in the case of fourth-degree hemorrhoids or large symptomatic external hemorrhoids or troublesome skin tags, some degree of excision is going to be required. Clearly this will always be painful, as operating in entirely insensate skin and mucosa is impossible with excision of an external component.

The Milligan-Morgan procedure as originally described appears to be flawed in terms of its anatomical basis. It really only addresses the external component properly, and, as Parks points out, it involves ligation of the pedicle in a sensate part of the anal canal. In reality most surgeons do not perform the operation as originally described and would ligate the pedicle higher up in the anal canal where it is insensate.

Unfortunately, the Ferguson closed hemorrhoidectomy [2] has never been compared to the Parks operation in a randomized clinical trial. In Ferguson's original description he stresses the importance of making elliptical incisions around both the internal and external components, thus removing very little anoderm at the dentate line and allowing the anoderm to be closed easily by a continuous suture. In more recent descriptions the same point has been made by describing the incision as "hourglass" in shape. All descriptions talk of the importance of undermining the resulting flaps of anoderm to remove residual submucosal hemorrhoidal tissue not already excised. Thus Ferguson's technique is really similar to Parks's except that the redundant mucosa and anoderm of the internal and external hemorrhoids are removed.

There is much overlap between the various techniques of hemorrhoidectomy and few surgeons practice the techniques exactly as originally described, making comparisons difficult. Parks's advice was that hemorrhoidectomy should minimize the removal of anoderm and rectal mucosa to avoid strictures. He also stressed the importance of avoiding ligating the pedicle within the sensate part of the anal canal to minimize pain. Regardless of whether one chooses to leave the wounds open or to close them, to excise mucosa and anoderm or to create flaps, Parks's advice should be followed as much today as in 1956.

References and Further Reading

1. Hosch SB, Knoefel WT, Pichlmaier U et al. Surgical treatment of piles. Dis Colon Rectum 1998;41:159–64.
2. Ferguson J, Heaton J. Closed haemorrhoidectomy. Dis. Colon Rectum 1959;2:176–79.
3. Filingeri V, Gravante G, Baldessari E et al. Prospective randomised trial of submucosal haemorrhoidectomy with radiofrequency bistoury vs. conventional Parks' operation. Tech Coloproctol 2004;8:31–36.
4. Milito G, Cortese F. The surgical treatment of haemorrhoids, 1st ed. Springer-Verlag, London 2002:93–96.
5. Parks A. The surgical treatment of haemorrhoids. Br J Surg 1956;43:337–51.
6. Roe A, Bartolo D, Vellacott K, Locke-Edmunds J, Mortensen N. Submucosal versus ligation excision haemorrhoidectomy: a comparison of anal sensation, anal sphincter manometry, and postoperative pain and function. Br J Surg 1987;74:948–51.
7. Rosa G, Lolli P, Piccinelli D, Vicenzi L et al. Submucosal reconstructive haemorrhoidectomy (Parks' operation): a 20-year experience. Tech Coloproctol 2005;9: 209–15.

14 Stapled Hemorrhoidopexy

Donato F. Altomare

Introduction

The search for a less painful operation for treating hemorrhoids has always been a major concern for colorectal surgeons, and stapled hemorrhoidopexy has represented an important step in this direction. The possibility of using a circular stapler in the treatment of hemorrhoids was first proposed by Allegra in 1990 [1], but the originality of Longo's procedure [2] lay in his proposal to treat hemorrhoids by resecting a circular ring of prolapsed mucosa above the dentate line rather than completely removing the hemorrhoids.

Since its introduction into clinical practice in 1998, stapled hemorrhoidopexy (SH) has divided coloproctologists, opposing those who favor this new technical approach in any clinical situation to those who are against it, a priori, in all situations. In the middle there is a wiser category of surgeons who prefer to appraise the best treatment for different clinical presentations of hemorrhoids and to use all the arrows available to the coloproctologist's bow, selecting the best option for the individual patient.

Since 1997 about 550,000 patients have been treated with stapled hemorrhoidopexy worldwide (personal communication by Ethicon EndoSurgery SpA) and more than 270 papers have been indexed in MEDLINE, confirming the high interest around the world in this new treatment.

Theoretical Basis of the Procedure

Based on Thompson's theory [3], this procedure aims to lift the hemorrhoid tissue into the upper anal canal, preventing further prolapse during straining, by resecting and stapling a circumferential band of prolapsed rectal mucosa above the hemorrhoids. An additional tip is closure by stapler stitches of the terminal branches of the rectal arteries, causing a reduction of the blood flow. Furthermore, the repositioning of the hemorrhoids in a low pressure zone of the anal canal allows a better upward drainage of the blood and shrinkage of the hemorrhoids. Most importantly, the suture line should be applied to the rectal mucosa, which lacks somatic innervation, thus causing only minor postoperative pain. The distal anal mucosa and the anal skin, with its valuable sensitivity, is spared.

The Matter of the Name of the Procedure

Several names have been proposed for this technique, ranging from the original "stapled hemorrhoidectomy," to "stapled anopexy," "circumferential stapled mucosectomy," and "procedure for prolapsing hemorrhoids (PPH)."

I. Khubchandani et al. (eds.), *Surgical Treatment of Hemorrhoids*, DOI 10.1007/978-1-84800-314-9_14,

After a consensus conference, the term stapled hemorrhoidopexy (SH) was deemed the most appropriate to describe the technique.

Indications

As with other surgical techniques, the best indications for SH have become clear only after unsuccessful or disappointing results were obtained for some of them. At the beginning the technique was used for all degrees of hemorrhoids except the first. Nowadays, almost all colorectal surgeons agree that the best indication for stapled hemorrhoidopexy is the third-degree hemorrhoidal prolapse, since the second can be successfully treated by less invasive techniques like rubber band ligation, and the fourth degree, despite some positive experiences, cannot be effectively corrected because of the absence of mobility of the prolapse [4].

Special Indications

This procedure has been successfully and safely applied in selected cases of rectal varices secondary to portal hypertension. Furthermore, some personal experiences have been reported in patients with coagulation problems and immuno-impairment.

Special considerations should be given to patients practicing anal receptive intercourse (e.g., homosexuals) because of the potential hazard of wounds due to the presence of metal staples in the anus.

Device

Originally a Proximate® ILS 33 mm stapler (Ethicon EndoSurgery) was utilized, sometimes with the help of a Lone Star self retractor (Lone Star Medical Products Inc., Houston, TX, USA) to expose the anal mucosa and to avoid including the anal cushions in the stapler line [5]. Subsequently,

a dedicated kit was designed and patented. This included a modified 33 mm hemorrhoidal circular stapler (HCS33) a circular anal dilator (CAD33) a purse string suture anoscope (PSA33) and a suture threader (ST100), all included in the PPH01 kit of Ethicon Endo-Surgery. The stapler device was modified with regard to the shape of the head (made more conical), and the head became nonremovable. The case of the stapler was marked with a scale in cm and provided with two holes through which the sutures pass.

In 2003 a further option was introduced, in the form of a new version of the PPH03stapler, which is more ergonomic (having a shorter shaft that is easy to handle), with faster opening and closure. But the most important modification is the reduced height of the closure of the metal stitches (0.75 mm), which ensures better hemostasis.

Some variations of the technique have been described, using stapler devices and anal dilators produced by other companies (Tyco Healthcare and SapiMed), but they failed to achieve popularity. Very recently the PPH patent was copied in China, like many other devices, but at the moment this cheaper version of the PPH01 does not guarantee sufficient safety and reliability.

Surgical Technique

The patient is prepared as usual with a cleansing enema some hours before the procedure. A urinary catheter is not necessary, but can be used at the end of the procedure to empty the bladder in order to prevent urinary retention, particularly in male patients. Prophylactic antibiotics are not strictly necessary, as for most anal procedures, but could be used in patients at risk of infection. This point has been debated in the literature after the first case of severe sepsis after stapled hemorrhoidopexy [6] was described, but the utility of antibiotic prophylaxis in this procedure has never been proven in randomized controlled trials.

The patient is generally placed in the lithotomy position, although the prone jackknife position is preferred by some surgeons because it favors hemorrhoidal drainage and reduces bleeding. Epidural anesthesia is usually administered, although the procedure has been successfully performed under local anesthesia or perineal block [7].

The first step of the procedure involves positioning of four sutures (silk 0 for example) at the four cardinal points of the anal verge, then the anus is gently dilated with a lubricated finger and the prolapsed mucosa and hemorrhoids are repositioned within the anal canal with the help of a small piece of gauze. This procedure, together with a gentle traction of the sutures around the anus, facilitates the subsequent introduction of the CAD, which is then tied to the anal verge using the sutures already in place (Fig. 14.1).

After cleansing the rectum of any residual mucus or feces, the site for placement of the purse string should be identified; this is the most crucial point in the entire procedure. The transparent CAD enables the operator to control the position of the dentate line, which appears paler compared to the rest of the mucosa and is usually in the middle of the CAD. A further 2 cm of the proximal anal canal are generally covered and protected by the CAD; this means that the internal anal sphincter should be entirely protected by the CAD. After introduction of the purse string suture anoscope, the site for the purse string is identified about 2–3 cm proximally to the edge of the CAD (rectal mucosa), 4–5 cm from the dentate line. The purse string is fashioned clockwise by applying 0 or 2/0 Prolene sutures symmetrically around the entire circumference (Fig. 14.2). Care should be taken, mainly in women, to avoid including the vaginal

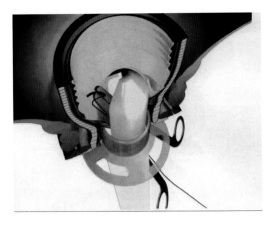

Figure 14.2 A 2/0 Prolene suture on 30 mm curve needle is used for a purse string 2–3 cm from the edge of the CAD.

wall or the Douglas pouch anteriorly. The purse string suture anoscope should be retracted and reinserted into the anus after each passage of the suture to prevent any rotation of the mucosal folds. The purse string should include only mucosal and submucosal tissue, although accidental inclusion of a smooth muscle layer in the resected doughnut is very frequent. When the operation is performed correctly, however, this muscle tissue is found to belong to the low rectal internal muscle layer and not to the internal anal sphincter. Originally, Longo recommended preparing a purse string about 2 cm away from the dentate line and leaving some mucosa bridges for fear of causing stricture. On the contrary, it is now recommended to begin the next bite very close to the exit of the previous stitch in order to prevent any gap in the mucosa, which could lead to incomplete mucosal excision.

At this point the purse string suture anoscope is retracted and the stapler introduced through the completely opened anoscope, placing the anvil well beyond the purse string. Attention should be paid not to close the purse string inadvertently before positioning the head of the stapler proximal to it. The suture is then gently pulled and tied around the stapler shaft (Fig. 14.3). The loose ends of the suture are extracted through the stapler casing channel using the suture threader.

Applying appropriate traction, the mucosa is pulled into the chamber of the casing while the

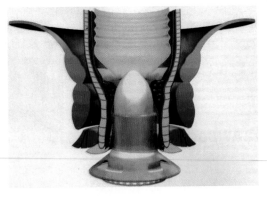

Figure 14.1 A well-lubricated CAD33 is gently inserted into the anus without sphincter stretch.

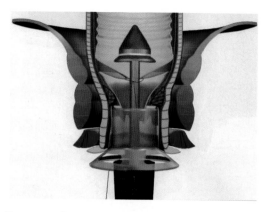

Figure 14.3 After the introduction of the opened PPH03 into the anus, the purse string is tied around the shaft and the prolapsed mucosa accommodates into the case of the PPH03.

procedure must be carried out very diligently, since postoperative bleeding occurs as a result of an incomplete hemostasis at the staple line. Usually some 3/0 Vycril sutures are necessary to achieve complete hemostasis. The use of a hemostatic sponge is rarely necessary. At the end of the operation a 22 french Foley catheter is inserted into the anus and blown up with 20–30 ml of water. Rectal lavage is then performed until the rinsing water is completely free of blood. The catheter is left in place for some hours (or overnight) to detect any postoperative bleeding, and if necessary, to treat by gentle traction on the inflated balloon. The use of local anesthetic infiltration of the staple line through the mucosa or externally is advocated by some surgeons to decrease postoperative pain.

stapler is closed. It is important to keep the stapler aligned along the axis of the anal canal and to look at the centimeter scale on the stapler casing, in order to control the position of the stapler in the anal canal. The closure of the stapler must be complete and maintained for a few seconds. The stapler is then fired after removal of the safety catch (Fig. 14.4). The stapler cannot be retracted unless it is slightly opened by one or two rounds. The resected specimen should be inspected after its removal from the casing chamber.

The suture line is then carefully inspected to detect any bleeding spots. This step of the

Double Purse String Technique

The use of a double purse string was originally proposed by Longo [2] in cases of mucosal prolapse exceeding 3 cm. Although not popular, this variation of the technique is preferable in my experience, since it enables a large amount of the mucosal prolapse to be resected and can better correct asymmetrical hemorrhoidal prolapse. This is necessary, for example, when one quadrant of the anal mucosa is prolapsed more than others. The two purse strings should be parallel or not, according to the symmetry of the prolapse and should be placed 1–2 cm apart. They should be started at 12 and 6 o'clock in order to be able to extract the sutures through the stapler casing channel using the appropriate suture threader.

A recent randomized controlled trial on single versus double purse string in stapled hemorrhoidopexy has confirmed this view, showing that the double purse string can yield better hemostasis and a larger amount of resected mucosa [8].

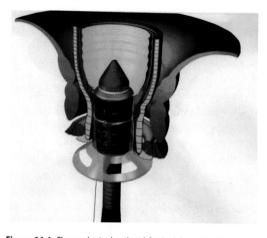

Figure 14.4 The stapler is closed and fired while maintaining a moderate traction on the threads.

Drawbacks and Complications

Despite some obvious advantages of stapled over conventional hemorrhoidectomy, this technique is still encountering some difficulty in gaining the expected widespread popularity, and even the meta-analyses carried out on this topic have reported inconsistent results. The major drawbacks of stapled hemorrhoidopexy are:

1. the increased cost of the procedure;
2. rare, but severe, complications; and
3. recurrence of the prolapse.

Cost of the Procedure

In times of healthcare restrictions in all western nations, the advantages of adopting a new, more expensive technique need to be well documented. Although the advantage of minor postoperative pain is of paramount importance for patients, it has only indirect economic effects, in terms of a more rapid return to work. Some studies have documented the feasibility of performing stapled hemorrhoidopexy as a day case procedure, even under local anesthesia [9], but the fear of possible early complications has prevented the diffusion of SH as a day surgery procedure.

Complications

At the beginning of the experiences with SH the major fears among coloproctologists were the occurrence of postoperative bleeding, rectal strictures, or fecal incontinence. Postoperative bleeding can occur from the suture line, having a comparable frequency rate to closed hemorrhoidectomy (CH) (about 5% or less) [10], but unlike bleeding after CH, the blood can collect in the rectum and sigmoid colon leading to severe anemia and even shock before the bleeding becomes clinically evident. For this reason, a gauze (or better, a Foley catheter) is placed in the rectum in the immediate postoperative period to detect early bleeding. Such early bleeding can be treated safely with endorectal compression by means of an intrarectal balloon, using a large Foley catheter inflated with 30–40 ml of water. Reoperation is rarely required. The occurrence of rectal stricture at the stapler line has very rarely been recorded [21], and the risk of fecal incontinence is negligible [11] if the technique is performed properly in patients without previous sphincter damage. In

this regard, care must be paid, particularly in multiparous women, even if asymptomatic, because the anal sphincter could already have been damaged by vaginal deliveries.

Another very common early complication is fecal urgency. Although the reason for this problem has not been fully elucidated, edema at the suture line, together with a potential reduction of rectal compliance, can play a role. Fecal urgency usually lasts a few weeks but in rare cases has been described even after one year.

Severe postoperative pain can occur, albeit in less than 5% of cases [12]. Although in most of these cases a fault in the operative procedure is clearly evident (low placement of the stapler line, involvement of the puborectalis muscle fibers), in rare cases there is no evident reason (variations in the somatic innervation have been postulated).

Besides these relatively common complications, a number of severe, sometimes life-threatening complications have been described. Although the incidence is low, the severity of these complications is extremely worrying and the medico-legal consequences for the surgeon are devastating. Some of these complications are new and specific to this operation and their treatment is neither standardized nor easy.

It has been objected that even after CH or minor anal procedures like rubber band ligation or sphincterotomy, some of these life-threatening complications have arisen, yet all these procedures have been performed for decades on millions of patients.

Septic complications are rare following hemorrhoidectomy and for this reason the use of prophylactic antibiotics is not recommended by the ASCRS. But for SH there is a tendency in several centers to use antibiotics, since some cases of rectal perforation, severe generalized sepsis [13], Fournier gangrene [14], and even death have been described.

Other severe complications like rectovaginal fistulas [15], rectal pocket syndrome, intramural hematoma, rectal occlusion [16], and obstructed defecation due to sandglass deformation of the rectal ampulla are clearly attributable to surgical inexperience and mistakes; but, nevertheless, they are very difficult to mend, even in the hands of experienced colorectal surgeons.

Recurrence

Although there is still no certainty in the literature about this matter, a higher recurrence rate compared to CH could be expected for at least two reasons. First of all, the operation may not be performed properly, and if there is insufficient resected mucosa, the use of a second stapler during the same operation is never considered because of the cost of the procedure. Secondly, the amount of prolapse is sometimes excessive compared with the space available in the stapler case and so only a part of the prolapse can be resected. This means that in most cases it is a question of residual prolapse rather than recurrence. Finally, SH cannot cure external hemorrhoids which will persist after this procedure due to their vascular supply from pudendal pedicles.

Comparison with Other Techniques

Many prospective randomized trials have been reported so far in the international literature comparing SH with the most widely applied technique, the Milligan-Morgan Hemorrhoidectomy (MMH) or Ferguson operation. The results of these studies have been analyzed in four meta-analyses or systematic reviews [17, 18, 19, 20], and one Cochrane review [21] but with inconsistent results. In fact, different points of view are presented. Two of these studies [17, 19]underlined the short term benefits of reduced pain and early return to working activities, although the lack of reported follow-up prevented any definite conclusions from being drawn about its efficacy compared to CH. Another review [18] mainly focused on the risk of severe complications, and others underlined the problem of hemorrhoids recurrence, reported to be significantly higher after SH in the Cochrane review of 2006 but equivalent to conventional hemorrhoidectomy in the latest metanalysis produced in 2007 [20].

The uncertainty still present about the true role and safety of SH can be seen by looking at the different conclusions reported in these metanalyses:

- Stapled hemorrhoidopexy may be at least as safe as conventional hemorrhoidal surgical techniques; however the efficacy of PPH compared with MMH could not be determined (Sutherland Arch Surg 2002).
- "PPH has unique potential complications and is a less effective cure compared with hemorrhoidectomy. It may be offered to patients seeking a less painful alternative to conventional surgery" (Nisar, DCR 2004).
- PPH may be at least as safe as MMH; however, the efficacy of PPH compared with MMH could not be determined absolutely (Lan P, Colorectal Dis 2006).
- Stapled hemorrhoidopexy is associated with a higher long-term risk of hemorrhoid recurrence and the symptom of prolapse. It is also likely to be associated with a higher likelihood of long-term symptom recurrence and the need for additional operations compared to conventional surgery (Jayaraman S, Cochrane Review 2007).
- PPH stapled hemorrhoidopexy is safe with many short-term benefits. The long-term results are similar to those using conventional procedures (Tjiandra, DCR 2007).

Stapled hemorrhoidopexy has also been compared with other hemorrhoidal procedures which are claimed to be less painful, like rubber band ligation, transanal hemorrhoidal arteries Doppler ligation (THD) [22], and the same Milligan-Morgan procedure using radiofrequency [23] or harmonic scalpel [24] instead of diathermy; but the data so far available are still uncertain and preliminary.

Long-Term Results

There is some confusion about the definition of "long-term," because it is not clear from the literature how long a time is needed to detect hemorrhoids recurrence. Few papers with a longer follow-up are available in the literature, two of which are long-term revisions of previously published papers.

In the study by Van de Stadt [25], after a mean follow-up of 46 months, recurrent or persistent symptoms of hemorrhoids were similar after CH and SH, although recurrent external prolapse requiring redo surgery was significantly higher after SH.

In the study by Au-Yong [26], at a follow-up of 42 months, the recurrence rate and functional results were similar in the two groups of patients. In the recent paper by Ganio et al. [27], after a mean follow-up of 84 months no differences in outcome were detected. However, it should be pointed out that all these papers were designed to detect a relevant reduction in postoperative pain, and therefore the sample size was calculated for this endpoint and not for recurrence, which would probably have required the recruitment of a larger number of patients. This makes these studies highly prone to a type 2 error.

Conclusions

After about 10 years of experience since the introduction of SH, some points are now clear to the colorectal surgeon. The ideal clinical indication for SH is third-degree internal hemorrhoids. The operation is less painful than the conventional excision procedure allowing for an earlier return to work, but in the long term, it poses a higher risk of recurrence of symptoms.

Both techniques can result in comparable postoperative bleeding, although after SH this complication may be more severe if not recognized quickly. Both techniques may result in rare but severe complications, but after SH they are probably more frequent and of a different nature.

References

1. Allegra G. Experiences with mechanical staplers: hemorrhoidectomy using a circular stapler. G Chir 1990; 11:95–97.
2. Longo A. Treatment of hemorrhoids disease by reduction of mucosa and hemorrhoidal prolapse with a circular suturing device: a new procedure. Proc 6th world congress of endoscopic surgery. Rome, Monduzzi Editore, Bologna 1998:777–84.
3. Thomson WH. The nature of haemorrhoids. Br J Surg 1975;62:542–52.
4. Altomare DF, Roveran A, Pecorella G et al. The treatment of hemorrhoids: guidelines of the Italian Society of Colorectal Surgery. Tech Coloproctol 2006;10:181–86.
5. Altomare DF, Rinaldi M, Chiumarulo C et al. Treatment of external anorectal mucosal prolapse with circular stapler: an easy and effective new surgical technique. Dis Colon Rectum 1999;42:1102–1105.
6. Molloy RG, Kingsmore D. Life threatening pelvic sepsis after stapled hemorrhoidectomy. Lancet 2000; 355(9206):810.
7. Esser S, Khubchandani I, Rakhmanine M. Stapled hemorrhoidectomy with local anesthesia can be performed safely and cost-efficiently. Dis Colon Rectum 2004;47:1164–69.
8. Perez-Vicente F, Arroyo A, Serrano P et al. Prospective randomised clinical trial of single versus double purse-string stapled mucosectomy in the treatment of prolapsed haemorrhoids. Int J Colorectal Dis 2006;21:38–43.
9. Ong CH, Chee Boon Foo E, Keng V. Ambulatory circular stapled haemorrhoidectomy under local anesthesia versus circular stapled haemorrhoidectomy under regional anaesthesia. ANZ J Surg 2005;75:184–86.
10. Ravo B, Amato A, Bianco V, Boccasanta P, Bottini C, Carriero A, Milito G, Dodi G, Mascagni D, Orsini S, Pietroletti R, Ripetti V, Tagariello GB. Complications after stapled hemorrhoidectomy: can they be prevented? Tech Coloproctol 2002;6:83–88.
11. Altomare DF, Rinaldi M, Sallustio PL et al. Long-term effects of stapled haemorrhoidectomy on internal anal function and sensitivity. Br J Surg 2001;88:1487–91.
12. Wexner SD. Persistent pain and fecal urgency after stapled haemorrhoidectomy. Tech Coloproctol 2001;5:56–57.
13. Pessaux P, Lermite E, Tuech JJ et al. Pelvic sepsis after stapled hemorrhoidectomy. J Am Coll Surg 2004; 199:824–825.
14. Bonner C, Prohm P, Storkel S. Fournier gangrene as a rare complication after stapler hemorrhoidectomy. Case report and review of the literature. Chirurg 2001;72:1464–66.
15. McDonald PJ, Bona R, Cohen CR. Rectovaginal fistula after stapled hemorrhoidopexy. Colorectal Dis 2004;6:64–65.
16. Stukavec J, Horak L. Complications of the Longo procedure—rectal occlusion. Rozhl Chir 2006;85:517–19.
17. Sutherland LM, Burchard AK, Matsuda et al. A systematic review of stapled hemorrhoidectomy. Arch Surg 2002; 137:1395–406.
18. Nisar PJ, Acheson AG, Neal KR, Scholefield JH. Stapled hemorrhoidopexy compared with conventional hemorrhoidectomy: systematic review of randomized, controlled trials [review]. Dis Colon Rectum 2004;47:1837–45.
19. Lan P, Wu X, Zhou X, Wang J, Zhang L. The safety and efficacy of stapled hemorrhoidectomy in the treatment of hemorrhoids: a systematic review and meta-analysis of ten randomized control trials. Int J Colorectal Dis 2006;21:172–78.
20. Tjandra JJ, Chan MK. Systematic review on the procedure for prolapse and hemorrhoids (stapled hemorrhoidopexy) [review]. Dis Colon Rectum 2007;50:878–92.
21. Jayaraman S, Colquhoun PH, Malthaner RA. Stapled versus conventional surgery for hemorrhoids. Cochrane DB Syst Rev 2006;18:CD005393.

22. Tagariello C, Dal Monte PP, Sarago M. Doppler-guided transanal hemorrhoidal dearterialisation. Chir Ital 2004; 56:693–97.
23. Basdanis G, Papadopoulos VN, Michalopoulos A, Apostolidis S, Harlaftis N. Randomized clinical trial of stapled hemorrhoidectomy vs. open with Ligasure for prolapsed piles. Surg Endosc 2005;19:235–39.
24. Chung CC, Cheung HY, Chan ES et al. Stapled hemorrhoidopexy vs. harmonic scalpel hemorrhoidectomy: a randomized trial. Dis Colon Rectum 2005;48:1213–19.
25. Van de Stadt J, D'Hoore A, Duinslaeger M et al. Belgian Section of Colorectal Surgery, Royal Belgian Society for Surgery. Long-term results after excision haemorrhoidectomy versus stapled haemorrhoidopexy for prolapsing hemorrhoids; a Belgian prospective randomized trial. Acta Chir Belg 2005;105:44–52.
26. Au-Young I, Rowsell M, Hemingway DM. Randomised controlled clinical trial of stapled haemorrhoidectomy vs conventional haemorrhoidectomy: a three and a half year follow up. Colorectal Dis 2004;6:37–38.
27. Ganio E, Altomare DF, Milito G et al. Long-term outcome of a multicentre randomized clinical trial of stapled haemorrhoidopexy versus Milligan-Morgan haemorrhoidectomy. Br J Surg 2007;94:1033–37.

15 "Total" Hemorrhoidectomy: The Whitehead Hemorrhoidectomy and Modifications

Mattias Soop and Bruce G. Wolff

Introduction

The concept of removing "the complete ring of pile-bearing mucous membrane" was introduced by Manchester surgeon Walter Whitehead in 1882 [1], and five years later he published his personal series of 300 patients [2]. The total hemorrhoidectomy described by Whitehead suffered early criticism due to a high incidence of complications reported by others using his technique. Favorable outcomes have been reported, however, by many authors employing both Whitehead's original procedure and its modifications. Today, 125 years after its description, the concept of total hemorrhoidectomy still prevails in many centers.

The fundamental difference between total hemorrhoidectomy and more traditional hemorrhoidectomies (such as the Milligan-Morgan or the Ferguson operations) is that the entire segment of dilated anal cushions and its overlying mucosa (and in some descriptions, skin) is circumferentially excised, rather than single hemorrhoids being selectively excised. It follows that the indication for total hemorrhoidectomy is circumferential, converging piles, where a traditional hemorrhoidectomy would leave a large amount of hemorrhoidal tissue behind.

The Original Whitehead Hemorrhoidectomy

The total hemorrhoidectomy described by Whitehead begins with an incision in the mucosa "at its junction with the skin round the entire circumference of the bowel" and the dissection of "the mucous membranes and attached hemorrhoids . . . from the submucous bed" [2]. Once the dissection has reached an area above the hemorrhoids, the mucosa is divided transversely and the specimen thus removed. The method of closure of the resulting circumferential wound has been the subject of much discussion and subsequent modifications. Whitehead clearly describes his method: "the free margin of the severed [mucous] membrane above is attached . . . to the free margin of the skin below" [2] (Fig. 15.1B).

In his report of his first 300 cases operated over 9 years, Whitehead reported that the mortality and short-term and long-term morbidity was nil [2]. The length and method of follow-up was not specified. His hemorrhoidectomy initially enjoyed immediate and wide popularity, as is apparent from the large number of studies published in the late 1890s and early 1900s. Although the results of the procedure in most hands were excellent, there were a few early authors who were highly critical. Kelsey in 1893 reported the first

I. Khubchandani et al. (eds.), *Surgical Treatment of Hemorrhoids*, DOI 10.1007/978-1-84800-314-9_15,

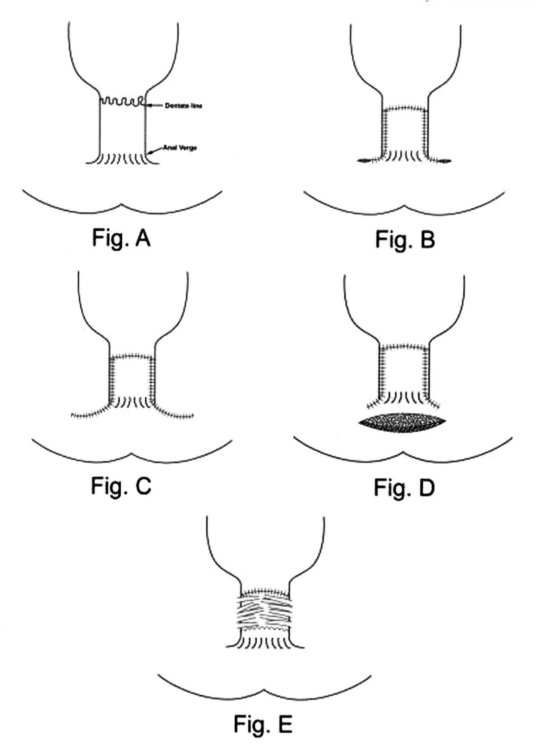

Figure 15.1 Schematic representation of the main modifications of the Whitehead hemorrhoidectomy. In **A**, normal anatomy is outlined. In **B**, the end result of the Buie modification is shown. Please note level of mucocutaneous suture line at or near normal level of dentate line. In **C**, the extended, radial relaxing incisions of the Fansler modification are shown. Figure **D** shows the sagittal relaxing incision of the Rand modification. The Granet modification, where the mucosal edge is sutured to underlying muscle rather than to the cutaneous edge, is shown in **E**.

case of mucosal ectropion (or so-called wet anus, or Whitehead deformity) [3]. Andrews in 1895 published the findings of his questionnaire audit of results of the Whitehead hemorrhoidectomy among European and North American surgeons. In highly subjective phrasing, he reported a large number of cases with complications including mucosal ectropion, stenosis, incontinence, chronic pain, and even fatal peritonitis [4, 5].

What caused the wide variation in results among different authors? The problem may lie in a confusion at the time of Whitehead's writing regarding the level of the mucocutaneous border, as demonstrated in detail by Bonello in 1988 [6], but pointed out previously in 1945 by DeCourcy [7]. Today, the mucocutaneous border is universally understood to be at the dentate line. Bonello demonstrated, however, that medical writing in the late 1800s and early 1900s often defined the mucocutaneous border at the intersphincteric line, some 3–20 mm distal to the dentate line [6]. This may explain the "disastrous" results of the Whitehead hemorrhoidectomy in some hands. It is ironic that Whitehead specifically stressed the importance of making the distal incision "through the mucous membrane and not through the skin," avoiding excision of any anoderm [2] (Fig. 15.1B). It seems inappropriate, therefore, that mucosal ectropion should be referred to as "Whitehead deformity."

The Modified Whitehead Hemorrhoidectomies

While the Whitehead operation nearly disappeared from the literature following the critical reports cited above, a number of modified circumferential or total hemorrhoidectomies were described from the 1930s until modern times. Several "modified" procedures differed very little from Whitehead's operation; indeed some differed only in the perioperative care. There are, however, three modifications of Whitehead's method of total hemorrhoidectomy which differ significantly from the original operation and have been described in some detail. All three modifications emphasize the

avoidance of mucosal ectropion by the avoidance of a distal mucocutaneous suture line near or at the anal verge. The method by which this is achieved differs between the three modifications.

Anodermal Advancement Flaps

Louis A Buie Sr of the Mayo Clinic described a modification in 1932 in which the anoderm, rather than merely being preserved as Whitehead emphasized, is undermined and then advanced cephalad as four separate flaps to meet the mucosal incision line to which it is sutured without tension [8]. This ensures that the dentate line is recreated at or slightly above the level of the normal dentate line (Fig. 15.1B and Fig. 15.2). Details of the procedure and reported outcomes will be discussed in more detail below.

Relaxing Incisions

Fansler of the Minneapolis group in 1933 published a modification which was very similar to the Buie modification, with the addition of longer, radiating linear incisions in the perianal skin, rendering the undermined anodermal flaps more mobile [9] (Fig. 15.1C).

Another type of relaxing incision was proposed by Rand in 1969 [10]. Two 7–9 cm long sagittal relaxing incisions 3 cm lateral to the anus were suggested (Fig. 15.1D). No outcome data specifically evaluating the Fansler or the Rand modifications have been published.

Anodermal Skin Healing by Secondary Intention

Granet in 1953 proposed suturing the mucosal edge to the exposed subcutaneous tissue and lower edge of the internal sphincter, rather than to the anoderm [11] (Fig. 15.1E). This allows the surgeon to remove any external components without fear of mucosal ectropion. Granet claimed that the resulting circular open wound in the anal canal healed by granulation and resulted in a new epithelium of the

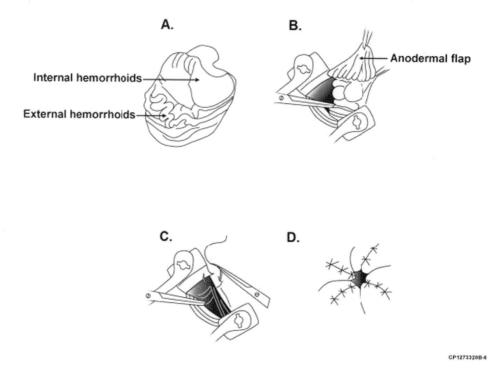

Figure 15.2 Key steps of the Buie modification of the Whitehead hemorrhoidectomy. In **A**, circumferential hemorrhoids are shown. In **B**, one quadrant is exposed by retractors and a rectangular or trapezoid anodermal flap is raised. The raised anodermal flap is the sutured to the mucosal edge at the level of the normal dentate line, **C**. The result is a circumferential suture line near or at the level of the normal dentate line, with the longitudinal suture lines visible only outside the anus, **D**. (Figure based on Fig. 15.1, Ref [13]. With kind permission of Springer Science and Business Media).

anal canal which eventually assumed the pliability and dilatability of the normal anoderm.

Although Granet did not provide any outcome data, a cohort of 41 consecutive patients operated upon with a technique identical to Granet's modification was presented in 1979 [12]. Long-term outcomes were favorable with no recurrences, stenosis in two patients, ectropion in one, and incontinence in one.

The Buie Modification of Whitehead's Hemorrhoidectomy

Patient Selection

Total hemorrhoidectomy removes a circumferential segment of hemorrhoidal tissue and overlying mucosa, and should therefore be reserved for nearly or completely circumferential hemorrhoids. Relative contraindications include a thin and tight anoderm, chronic diarrhea of any etiology, proctitis, anal incontinence, and late (>24 h) incarceration or strangulation.

Technique

The operation may be performed as an outpatient procedure in local patients. One tap water enema is usually sufficient to achieve a clear operative field. The operation is carried out in general or spinal anesthesia with the patient in the prone-jackknife position with the buttocks taped apart. The advantages of this position far outweigh the disadvantages, and include proper exposure and bleeding away from the operative field.

A Smith-Buie retractor is used for exposure. An anodermal flap extending approximately 3 cm in the cephalad-caudal direction and extending across a lateral portion of the circumference of the anal canal is first raised. This is done by incision of a rectangular or trapezoidal flap of anoderm which is undermined with curved, double-pointed operating scissors (Fig. 15.2B). Cephalad to this flap, a similar section of mucosa is excised, along with all adherent hemorrhoidal tissue. The anodermal flap is then advanced up the anal canal where it is sutured to the free edge of the mucosa, catching small bites in the internal sphincter, by a monofilament absorbable continuous suture. The dentate line is thus recreated at or slightly above the level of the natural dentate line (Fig. 15.1B).

This procedure is repeated circumferentially with a total of four flaps. Skin bridges may be left between flaps unless hemorrhoidal tissue would be left by doing so. Relaxing incisions are not necessary. The only suture lines visible outside the anus will be the four longitudinal suture lines, connecting the four flaps (Figs. 15.1B and 15.2D). Small draining openings may be left distally (as in Fig. 15.1B).

A rubber dam with haemostatic dressing is inserted in the anal canal and removed later the same day prior to discharge. Patients are instructed to take 20-min sitz baths three times daily. Oral analgesics and a bulking agent or a stool softener are provided. Stimulant laxatives are avoided as they may cause liquid stool persistently spilling over the suture line. Office workers can return to work after one week, while manual laborers often need three weeks off work.

Published Outcomes

Burchell in 1976 published a cohort series of 179 patients who underwent a modified Whitehead hemorrhoidectomy identical to the Buie modification. Patients were followed up by questionnaires. No mucosal ectropion and no recurrence were noted in this series.

The Mayo Clinic experience of the Buie modification of Whitehead's hemorrhoidectomy has been reported in detail. Culp reported outcomes of his 556 patients operated upon between 1963

and 1983 [13]. Follow up for three years was complete for 440 patients. Although the flap dehisced in 7% of patients, only 1% had infections and all wounds but one eventually healed. No recurrence or mucosal ectropion occurred in this series.

Similar findings were reported by Sagar for 110 patients who underwent the procedure between 1984 and 1993 [14]. Flap dehiscence occurred in 3%. Anal stenosis was observed in 6% of patients in this study, but all responded well to simple anal dilatation. Again, no recurrences or mucosal ectropion occurred. These outcomes compared favorably to those of a gender- and age-matched group of patients who were operated upon by closed Ferguson hemorrhoidectomy, where 3% needed a further hemorrhoidectomy procedure. The prevalence of postoperative urinary retention was 25% in the modified Whitehead group, vs. 15% in the control group. This may reflect a higher degree of postoperative pain after total hemorrhoidectomy than after traditional surgery, highlighting the importance of adequate postoperative analgesia.

Discussion

Total hemorrhoidectomy retains its place in modern hemorrhoid surgery as an option for large, circumferential hemorrhoids. The authors favor the Buie modification of the Whitehead hemorrhoidectomy. This method recreates the dentate line at a natural level in the anal canal and removes all hemorrhoidal tissue, thus minimizing complications as well as recurrences, as reported in large case series.

An additional benefit of this operation, in the context of a teaching institution, is that the dissection in the Buie modification of the Whitehead hemorrhoidectomy is essentially the same dissection used for repair of keyhole deformities or ectropions, the excision of small anal verge cancers, anoplasty, and the mucosal excision preformed before hand-sewn ileoanal pouch anastomosis.

References

1. Whitehead W. The surgical treatment of hemorrhoids. Br Med J 1882;1:148–150.
2. Whitehead W. Three hundred consecutive cases of hemorrhoids cured by excision. Br Med J 1887;1:449–451.
3. Kelsey CB. Diseases of the rectum and anus: their pathology, diagnosis, and treatment. New York: William Wood & Co., 1893.
4. Andrews E. Some of the evils caused by Whitehead's operation and by its modification, the American operation. Trans Illinois Med Soc 1895;433.
5. Andrews E. Disastrous results following Whitehead's operation for piles and the so-called American operation. Columbus Med J 1895;15:97.
6. Bonello JC. Who's afraid of the dentate line? The Whitehead hemorrhoidectomy. Am J Surg 1988;156:182–186.
7. DeCourcy JL. Whitehead operation for hemorrhoids. Cincinnati J Med 1945;25:490–494.
8. Buie LA. Proctoscopic examination and treatment of hemorrhoids and anal pruritus. Philadelphia: W B Saunders, 1932.
9. Fansler WA, Anderson JA. A plastic operation for certain types of hemorrhoids. J Am Med Assoc 1933;101:1064–1066.
10. Rand AA. The sliding skin-flap graft operation for hemorrhoids: a modification of the Whitehead procedure. Dis Colon Rectum 1969;12:265–276.
11. Granet E. An anorectoplasty for extensive and complicated hemorrhoids. Surgery 1953;34:72–87.
12. Barrios G, Khubchandani M. Whitehead operation revisited. Dis Colon Rectum 1979;22:330–332.
13. Wolff BG, Culp CE. The Whitehead hemorrhoidectomy. An unjustly maligned procedure. Dis Colon Rectum 1988;31:587–590.
14. Sagar PM, Wolff BG. The use of the modified Whitehead procedure as an alternative to the closed Ferguson hemorrhoidectomy. Tech Coloproctol 1999;3:131–134.

16 Pre-, Peri-, and Postoperative Management

Indru Khubchandani and Ramaz Metreveli

Preoperative Management

Inasmuch as hemorrhoidectomy is performed as outpatient surgery, generally with local anesthesia and sedation, minimal preoperative testing (PAT) is required. The patient is directed to interview with the anesthesia department prior to surgery. Unless comorbidities are present, a chest X-ray is not necessary. An electrocardiogram (EKG) is performed only in patients over 50 years of age. No laboratory tests are required, and a coagulation profile is necessary only if the patient has a prior history of bleeding.

Initially, the patient reports to the surgical suite after self-administration of a phospho-soda enema 2 h prior to the procedure. The patient will have had a regular meal the evening before and nothing per mouth after midnight. Any sedation before transportation to the operating room is left to the discretion of the anesthesiologist.

Perioperative Management

A patient scheduled for a hemorrhoidectomy may be facing the experience of surgery for the first time in his or her life. Unlike other aspects of medicine, there are very few mass media resources that publicize anorectal diseases or serve as references. During the initial preoperative visit there is not always enough time to allow for explanation of every detail of the postoperative course. In addition, the patient may not remember every detail that is provided. Therefore, it is critically important that the verbal information be supported by clearly written instructions or even a videotaped presentation.

Post-hemorrhoidectomy instructions should contain information regarding what the patient might expect in the immediate postoperative period and how to deal with possible complications. Topics addressed should include management of pain, wound care, ways of maintaining adequate bowel function, diet, and levels of physical activity, including return to work (Fig. 16.1). Potential complications, such as excessive pain, urinary retention, and bleeding should also be discussed.

Postoperative Care

Postoperative wound management varies from surgeon to surgeon. Many surgeons use dressing or even packing in the anal canal after hemorrhoidectomy. Routine use of packing is not recommended and rarely necessary for hemostatic purposes; it is uncomfortable and can also precipitate urinary retention. No intra-anal hemostatic packing is necessary. It is our practice to use a small Tefla® piece only, on the exterior of the wounds.

In addition to analgesics, sitz baths provide excellent wound care. Sitting in either a bathtub or a small

I. Khubchandani et al. (eds.), *Surgical Treatment of Hemorrhoids*, DOI 10.1007/978-1-84800-314-9_16,
© Springer-Verlag London Limited 2009

INSTRUCTIONS FOLLOWING ANORECTAL OPERATION

DIET
Resume your normal diet. We encourage you to have some roughage with each meal. Avoid hot/spicy foods and beer and wine, as these may cause irritation about the anus. We caution you not to drink alcohol while taking pain medications.

SITZ BATHS
Begin sitz baths the day of surgery – three times daily and after each bowel movement (5-15 minutes of bath water temperature). You may use the tub if the sitz bath itself is uncomfortable. More frequent usage is encouraged if anal discomfort warrants. Make only normal efforts to pass a stool. There may be false urges to defecate after meals, just walk away if nothing happens – the sitz bath is useful if you have these sensations and can help also if you have difficulty urinating. If you cannot urinate and feel uncomfortable, call the office.

DRESSING
Remove the outer dressing tonight. If there is a dressing **inside** the anus leave it in place. If this dressing is extruding the day after surgery, then it may be removed with a slight "tug", but if it is resistant then leave it in place as it will dissolve or fall out in the sitz bath.

PERSONAL HYGIENE
You may use toilet tissue as soon as tolerated. Baby wipes are a soft alternative.

MEDICATIONS
Take Bisacodyl (laxative) tablets at bedtime -   __ Evening of surgery
          __ Day after surgery at bedtime

Citrucel is a bulk laxative, which increases the volume of stool through colon water retention, and may be started the day after surgery. Citrucel is a therapeutic fiber to supplement and complement roughage supplied by a proper diet of bran, fruits and vegetables. Take Citrucel as directed to achieve desired effect of regularity and comfort when attention should be directed towards your fiber intake. **If you have not had a bowel movement after the third day following surgery, take a Fleet enema or call the office.** Pain pills may be taken – one or two every 3-4 hours. These pills are narcotics and there may be a tendency to have dizziness or nausea. There are alternative medications if nausea persists.

GENERAL
Anorectal operations may vary with one, two, three, or more "rows" of stitches, or **none** at all. The doctor will discuss this with you. If you have stitches they will dissolve. In order for the stitches to dissolve, the tissues about the anus will create an inflammatory reaction, therefore, do not be alarmed by some soreness, bleeding, discharge, or false urges to defecate. Bleeding with the passage of stool is possible up to several weeks following surgery. If the bleeding is heavy and **does not stop** in a few minutes with gentle pressure (like when you cut yourself shaving), call us immediately. Do not be alarmed by swelling about the anus. These are not hemorrhoids, but simply due to the stitches. Strenuous exercise and heavy lifting are to be avoided for at least three weeks. You may drive when comfortable. Going up and down stairs should be limited if it causes discomfort.

See below for the date and time of your next appointment. Please call the office if you need to change the appointment. We will answer questions that may arise regarding work, sexual relations, diet, and physical activities. Insurance forms and work release can be handled at the office.

Figure 16.1 Postoperative instructions following hemorrhoidectomy.

pan containing warm water placed on the toilet provides excellent pain relief as well. Sitz baths can be started as early as the evening of the day of surgery. It is not necessary to add any soap, salts, or disinfectants to the water. It is our practice to provide the patient with a disposable sitz bath unit, which can be easily connected to household plumbing.

Activity and Diet

Activity should not be restricted after this type of anorectal surgery. Usually the most efficient limiting factor is the patient's pain control. The resumption of normal activity often accelerates healing and return of normal bowel function. Obviously, sports activities that can traumatize the perineum such as bicycle, horseback, or motorcycle riding should be avoided for several weeks after hemorrhoidectomy.

Restoration of adequate bowel function is especially important after hemorrhoidectomy. It is our practice to hand two tablets of Dulcolax® to the patient to be ingested the evening of surgery, to promote early bowel movement. It is important to encourage the patient to have a bowel movement whenever the urge occurs. A bowel movement that is delayed for several days may lead to hardening of the stool, since water is reabsorbed more intensively and the first bowel movement can lead to a trauma of a fresh wound with possible complications such as bleeding. The patient should be advised to have regular bowel movements as before surgery.

Bulk-forming laxatives such as pysllium and methylcellulose should be started in the preoperative or immediate postoperative period. Such agents produce a soft, bulky stool that is not traumatizing to the anal canal.

Postoperative Complications

Inadequate Pain Control

Anticipation of severe pain in the postoperative period is the most important reason why patients try to avoid hemorrhoidectomy as much as possible. It is well known that hemorrhoidectomy and tonsillectomy, surgical procedures on opposite sides of the gastrointestinal tract, are considered to be among the most painful. Complete elimination of pain after the hemorrhoidectomy is not realistic. Overly aggressive use of opioid narcotics may cause respiratory depression and decreased bowel function. Although some degree of pain is inevitable after hemorrhoidectomy, it is important to remember that severe pain out of proportion to findings on physical examination could be a sign of other sequelae. Sitz baths, as described above, are helpful in controlling pain. We favor oxycodone with acetaminophen (Percocet®, Endo Pharmaceuticals) as analgesia to be used at the patient's discretion.

Bleeding

A small amount of bleeding can occur after any type of hemorrhoidectomy, regardless if it was open or closed. It is very important to mention this during the preoperative counseling. Although six days was an average time period in our study [1], delayed bleeding can occur up to two weeks postoperatively. It is difficult to determine the exact amount of bleeding based on patients' observations via telephone. In these cases, it may become necessary to make arrangements to see the patient immediately in the office or the emergency room. Vital signs and hemoglobin levels should be obtained. Any symptoms of hypovolemia will require admission to the hospital for intravenous hydration and serial hemoglobin measurements.

Most cases of postoperative bleeding can be controlled in the office or emergency room. A Gelfoam® (Pfizer, Inc.) 100 pack, rolled as a tampon and wrapped with Surgicel® (Ethicon, Inc.) is introduced in the anal canal through an anoscope, only after the blood in the ampulla and the sigmoid colon is evacuated via a sigmoidscope, before insertion of the anoscope. Only very rarely is a trip to the operating room necessary, in order to identify and control the bleeding site by suture ligation. Excisional hemorrhoidectomy, dreaded over the years, can be performed safely and with controlled pain, if designed with appropriate preoperative counseling and postoperative management.

References

1. Rosen L, Sipe P, Stasik JJ, Riether RD, Trimpi HD. Outcome of delayed hemorrhage following surgical hemorrhoidectomy. Dis Colon Rectum 1993;36:743–746.

17 The Operative Treatment by, and Results of, Diathermy Hemorrhoidectomy

Kok-Yang Tan and Francis Seow-Choen

Introduction

Although many patients with symptomatic hemorrhoids may be successfully managed without surgery, there are still a large number of patients who require surgical excision of hemorrhoids. It is not uncommon for surgical excision of hemorrhoids to be associated with postoperative pain together with perianal discharge, itchiness, and irritation. The number of postoperative symptoms is highly variable, and depends on the severity of the hemorrhoidal disease, individual pain threshold, racial and cultural differences, quality and type of anesthesia, postoperative analgesia, and the surgical technique. Some of these factors are more important than others in influencing postoperative pain. For both surgeons and patients, it is important to know which surgical techniques have fewer postoperative complications and cause less pain.

Milligan-Morgan's open hemorrhoidectomy, in which the wound is left open, is commonly used in some parts of the world, while others prefer Ferguson's closed hemorrhoidectomy, in which the mucosa and skin are closed after removal of the hemorrhoids. Whitehead described a radical method for treatment of circumferential hemorrhoids. In all of these techniques, the dissection of the hemorrhoidal tissues was done originally using scissors, and the vascular pedicles were ligated. The use of diathermy was thought in the past to result in increased postoperative pain. The converse, however, is nearer the truth.

We use diathermy alone for the dissection and division of hemorrhoidal tissues. This may be adapted for all the different techniques of excisional hemorrhoidectomy that have been described thus far. The diathermy is set in a blend cut/coagulation mode for ease of dissection. A pointed diathermy tip is not essential in our experience.

Patients are placed in the lithotomy position and can be operated on under general, regional, or even local anaesthesia [1]. The perianal region and intersphincteric grooves are infiltrated with local anesthetic prior to dissection. Diathermy is used to dissect the hemorrhoidal tissue off the internal sphincter and the pedicle is secured using diathermy coagulation.

Postoperative care includes oral analgesics, topical 2% lignocaine jelly and adequate fluid intake. A micronized flavonidic fraction is usually given as well to reduce the risk of post-hemorrhoidectomy hemorrhage [2]. Postoperatively, toilet care must be by gentle showering with clean tap water. The use of toilet paper of whatever quality is positively discouraged.

Techniques of Diathermy Hemorrhoidectomy

Open Hemorrhoidectomy

This is an adaptation of the Milligan-Morgan method of open hemorrhoidectomy. After

I. Khubchandani et al. (eds.), *Surgical Treatment of Hemorrhoids*, DOI 10.1007/978-1-84800-314-9_17,
© Springer-Verlag London Limited 2009

displaying the hemorrhoidal tissue, the mucocutaneous junction is incised with diathermy. Each pedicle is dissected with diathermy to its apex above the dentate line, and excess hemorrhoidal tissue is amputated by diathermy after coagulation of the pedicle without transfixion suture or ligature. Adequate mucosal bridges must be preserved.

We compared the results of using scissors and diathermy for open hemorrhoidectomy [3]. Forty-nine consecutive patients with symptomatic prolapsed piles that were unsuitable for or had failed nonexcisional treatment were recruited into the study. They were randomized prospectively for conventional scissors excision with ligation or for diathermy excision. The median time for the surgery was 20 min (range 10–40 min) and 10 min (range 5–35 min) for scissors excision and diathermy groups, respectively ($P <0.05$). There was no statistically significant difference in the severity of postoperative pain between the two groups. However, the use of oral analgesics was significantly lower in the diathermy group ($P <0.02$).

The median length of follow-up was 35 weeks in both groups. Three patients in the scissors group and one patient in the diathermy group developed mild anal strictures, which were adequately treated by bulk laxatives alone. All wounds in both groups healed completely. There was no incidence of post-hemorrhoidectomy bleeding or anal incontinence in either group.

We concluded that diathermy excision of hemorrhoids was significantly faster than scissors excision, that there was no need for ligation of the vascular pedicles, and that there was a significant reduction in the oral analgesic requirements. The diathermy method does not cause any increase in early or late postoperative complications. Basis and Begrime [4] also arrived at the same conclusion when they compared the results of closed hemorrhoidectomy, open scissors (Milligan-Morgan) hemorrhoidectomy, and open diathermy hemorrhoidectomy without ligature of the pedicle. They studied 135 patients and found that open hemorrhoidectomy was associated with less postoperative pain and patients in the diathermy group used less analgesic. There also was no increased risk of postoperative hemorrhage in the group without pedicle ligation.

The use of the Harmonic Scalpel in excising hemorrhoids was also compared with diathermy by us [5]. Fifty patients were randomized to either diathermy or Harmonic Scalpel. There was no statistically significant difference in the operative time, pain scores, analgesia use, and complication rates between the two groups. Diathermy is thus not inferior to Harmonic Scalpel.

Closed Hemorrhoidectomy

The technique of using diathermy for dissection of hemorrhoids is also applicable to closed hemorrhoidectomy. We use a modified version of closed hemorrhoidectomy. Following adequate anesthesia, the hemorrhoidal columns are displayed. The hemorrhoidal tissues are then dissected free using diathermy. The vascular pedicle is then isolated individually and transfixed with an absorbable suture. The pedicle was then buried under the mucosa as the latter is closed. The reason for ligating the pedicle in closed hemorrhoidectomy is not to decrease postoperative hemorrhage, but to establish the first stitch for closing the mucosa.

We compared this technique prospectively in a randomized trial against closed hemorrhoidectomy using scissors dissection [6]. Both groups had 20 mls of 1:20,000 adrenaline in 0.5% bupivacaine infiltrated before surgery. Both groups had identical surgery, with the exception of the method of dissection of the hemorrhoidal tissues. All patients had three hemorrhoids removed. Forty-four patients underwent diathermy closed hemorrhoidectomy while 47 underwent closed hemorrhoidectomy using scissors excision. There was no statistically significant difference in the operating time between both groups. Pain score was assessed with a linear analogue scale by a blinded investigator.

The median pain scores were similar between the two groups throughout the first seven days. There was no statistical difference in the severity of postoperative pain. Those in the diathermy group required less oral analgesic over 7 days ($\underline{P} < 0.001$). However, intramuscular pethidine use was higher in the first 24 h after surgery in the diathermy group. There was no statistical difference in the use of lignocaine jelly or in the number of days to the first bowel movement. There were no differences in early or late postoperative complications, including post-hemorrhoidectomy bleeding, wound dehiscence, or anal stricture. We postulated that the pain from diathermy in the first day postoperatively may be due to edema from diathermy, but this improved rapidly to give less pain overall compared to scissors excision.

We also conducted a study between closed and open hemorrhoidectomy using diathermy in a prospective randomized trial [7]. Open hemorrhoidectomy was performed without ligation of the pedicle, while in closed hemorrhoidectomy, the pedicle was transfixed and the mucosal wound edges were sutured with absorbable sutures. Thirty-three patients underwent closed hemorrhoidectomy using diathermy and 34 patients underwent open hemorrhoidectomy using diathermy. There was no significant difference in the time taken to perform closed or open diathermy hemorrhoidectomy. There were also no differences in the postoperative pain score or analgesic requirement between the two groups. Patients with open hemorrhoidectomy had earlier bowel movements ($P < 0.001$) than closed hemorrhoidectomy patients; however, the length of time of hospitalization was not significantly different between the two groups.

There were also no differences in the incidence of postoperative bleeding or fecal impaction. However, complete wound healing took significantly longer after closed hemorrhoidectomy (mean [sem] 6.9 [0.7] weeks) compared with open hemorrhoidectomy (mean [sem] 4.9 [0.4] weeks) ($P < 0.05$). Although primary repair should lead to earlier wound healing in the closed hemorrhoidectomy group, this was not realized because of wound infection and dehiscence in eight patients after closed hemorrhoidectomy.

Parks [8] postulated that post-hemorrhoidectomy pain might be due to the exposed and denuded anal sphincter, resulting in anal spasm. He thus advocated closed or submucosal hemorrhoidectomy, claiming that pain is minimal following this technique. Other studies later showed that there was no improvement in pain scores following closed hemorrhoidectomy [9]. This was confirmed in our study.

Diathermy Coagulation

Diathermy coagulation to shrink and cause necrosis of the hemorrhoidal tissues is also used for the treatment of prolapsed hemorrhoids. In this method, a forceps is applied to the base of the hemorrhoid, ensuring that the tip is well above the dentate line. The forceps should lift the hemorrhoidal tissue off the underlying sphincter muscle. Monopolar diathermy on a high setting in coagulation mode is then applied to produce a visible white eschar, drawing in prolapsed anal mucosa.

A randomized trial comparing diathermy excision and diathermy coagulation for symptomatic, prolapsed hemorrhoids was performed [10]. Forty-five patients were randomized to undergo either diathermy excision or diathermy coagulation. There was no statistically significant difference in postoperative pain, analgesia use, and complication rates. However, diathermy coagulation tended to leave some residual skin components in patients with large prolapsed hemorrhoids.

Improving Outcome After Diathermy Hemorrhoidectomy

There is no doubt that postoperative spasm of the internal sphincter contributes to pain [11, 12]. As such there have been many modifications of surgical technique to decrease this spasm in attempts to reduce pain. Anal dilatation was used to reduce post-hemorrhoidectomy pain. However, this was associated with an increased risk of severe irreversible sphincter damage and anal incontinence. Internal anal sphincterotomy and suppositories have also been used but with little success [13, 14].

Topical glyceryl trinitrate (GTN) reduces anal canal pressures and improves anodermal blood flow [15, 16]. Post-hemorrhoidectomy topical use of GTN may reduce anal spasm and improve postoperative pain, while improved anodermal blood flow may accelerate wound healing. We conducted a randomized, prospective, double-blind placebo-controlled trial on 82 patients undergoing diathermy hemorrhoidectomy [17]. Patients were randomized to either 0.2% GTN ointment (Recto-gesic™, Cellegy Australia Pty Ltd, 203 New South Head Road, Edgecliff NSW 2027, Australia) or placebo (vaseline) ointment applied topically to the perianal region after open diathermy hemorrhoidectomy. Patients were asked to complete a postoperative pain diary. Wound healing was also assessed. Complete healing was defined as complete epithelialization of the wounds.

There were 40 patients in the GTN ointment arm and 42 patients in the placebo arm. There were no statistically significant differences in the sex, weight, type of hemorrhoid, type of surgery (emergency or elective), number of hemorrhoids excised, duration of surgery, hospital stay, and complication rate. Pain scores and analgesic usage were not significantly different. By week 3 however, 17 patients in the GTN arm had completely epithelialized wounds compared to 8 patients in the placebo arm ($P = 0.021$). Only 1 patient in the GTN arm experienced headaches requiring discontinuation of the ointment. We concluded that glyceryl trinitrate (0.2%) ointment is useful in improving the wound healing rates. However, pain reduction was not demonstrated in this study.

In another study, looking at the addition of methylene blue to local analgesics to prolong the postoperative local anesthetic effect, we found that methylene blue was effective in prolonging anesthesia for up to about 3 weeks [18]. We are currently using methylene blue in addition to local anesthesia for patients undergoing excision and hemorrhoidectomies and have found it to be an effective way of decreasing pain [18].

Special Circumstances

Circumferential Prolapsed Piles

The technique of diathermy for hemorrhoidectomy can also be used for circumferential prolapsed piles. The two common methods of

treatment of excisional circumferential prolapsed piles are modified radical hemorrhoidectomy and the four-pile hemorrhoidectomy [19]. Currently, Longo stapled hemorrhoidectomy is another alternative method of treating these sort of piles [20, 21]. Instead of using scissors dissection and ligation of the pedicles, we adapted the use of diathermy to both these methods.

For four-piles hemorrhoidectomy (Fig. 17.1), diathermy was used for excision of all three primary piles as previously described. The remaining largest secondary piles were then selected and dissected and excised using diathermy, without ligation of the pedicle. The mucocutaneous continuity of that pile was then restored using an absorbable suture.

For modified radical hemorrhoidectomy (Fig. 17.2), the anorectal mucosa was divided into three parts circumferentially and each third dealt with in turn. Artery forceps were applied to cause further prolapse of the normal rectal mucosa above the pile-bearing area and to put this third of the anorectal circumference on a stretch. Diathermy was used to make an incision above the dentate line. The mucosal flap was raised and freed from the underlying internal sphincter by diathermy. Grossly evident hemorrhoidal tissue and excess mucosa was then removed, taking care to avoid devascularization of the flap. The flap was then stitched to the proximal divided mucosal edge of the rectal mucosa and internal sphincter with an absorbable suture, thus pulling the anal skin and mucosa upwards into the anal canal. This level should be at or above the previous dentate line. This was repeated with the remaining two-thirds of the anal canal. On the occasion where flap tension was excessive, circumanal release incisions can be made as required.

We compared the above two techniques in a prospective randomized trial [19]. Twenty-eight patients with large third- or fourth-degree piles who were not suitable for the standard three-piles hemorrhoidectomy were recruited. Fourteen patients were randomized to radical hemorrhoidectomy and 14 to four-piles hemorrhoidectomy. The median duration of surgery was 30 min for the radical group and 10 min for the four-piles hemorrhoidectomy group ($P < 0.05$). Following healing of the

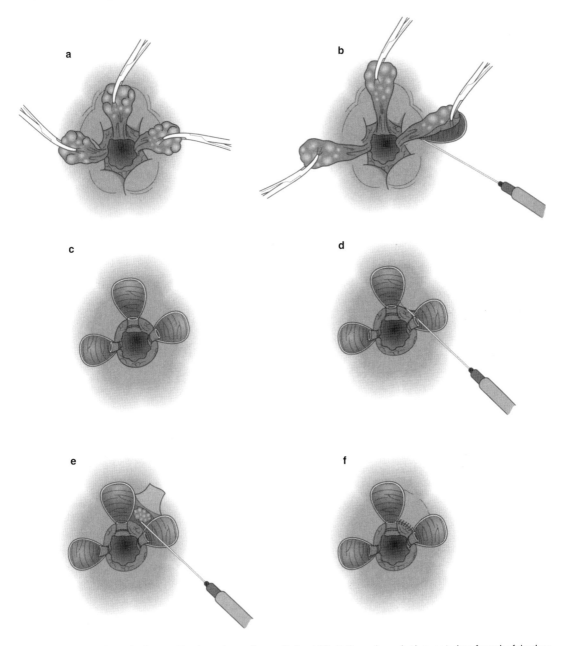

Figure 17.1 Four-pile hemorrhoidectomy. The three primary piles are displayed (**A**). Diathermy hemorrhoidectomy is done for each of the three primary piles (**B**). The three primary piles have been removed (**C**). The remaining largest secondary pile dissected (**D**) and excised (**E**). The mucocutaneous continuity restored (**F**).

hemorrhoidectomy wounds, all patients in the radical group were completely continent compared to 12 of 14 (85.7%) in the four-piles group. Two other patients (14.3%) in the four-piles group developed anal stricture requiring anal dilatation. Five patients in the radical hemorrhoidectomy group developed wound dehiscence that required secondary suture. Of these five patients, three developed anal stricture. Two patients had remnant anal skin tags in the radical group, compared to nine patients in the four-piles

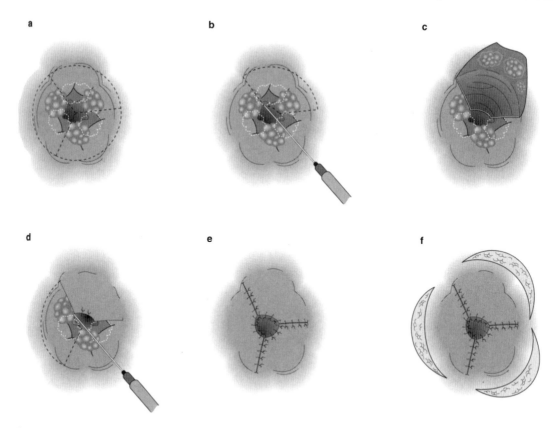

Figure 17.2 Modified radical hemorrhoidectomy. The anorectal mucosa was divided into three parts circumferentially (**A**). Incision made using diathermy above the dentate line (**B**). The mucosal flap was raised and freed from the underlying internal sphincter by diathermy (**C**). The flap was then stitched to the proximal divided mucosal edge of the rectal mucosa and internal sphincter with absorbable suture (**D**). After completion of remaining 2 parts (**E**). Circumanal release incisions made when flap tension was excessive (**F**).

group. Two of the patients in the four-pile group had residual symptomatic piles compared to none in the radical group.

At six months of follow-up, six patients in the 4 piles group considered the results to be excellent, seven acceptable and one was disappointed. In the radical group, two considered it to be excellent, ten acceptable and two were disappointed. Four-piles hemorrhoidectomy is much easier to perform than radical hemorrhoidectomy. Flap dehiscence is a problem with radical hemorrhoidectomy, occurring in 7.2–11.2% of cases. This resulted in a high incidence of anal stricture in the radical hemorrhoidectomy group, although there was no significant difference between the two groups in this study as far as anal stricture was concerned. Patient

satisfaction was better in the four-piles hemorrhoidectomy group, and this operation is preferred for circumferential prolapsed piles.

Acute Hemorrhoids

Acutely thrombosed, ulcerated, or gangrenous prolapsed hemorrhoids cause severe pain and disability to patients. It has been said that emergency hemorrhoidectomy is associated with an increased risk of portal pyemia, secondary hemorrhage, anal stenosis, and fecal incontinence. However, several studies [22, 23] have shown that emergency hemorrhoidectomy is safe and is an appropriate way of treating acute hemorrhoids.

We studied retrospectively 704 cases of hemorrhoidectomy done over a 24-month period [24]. All the cases of hemorrhoidectomy done in the last 8 months of the study were by diathermy without ligation of the hemorrhoidal pedicles. Five hundred elective cases and 204 emergency cases were evaluated for complications and functional results. The two groups were matched for age, sex, and race. Length of follow-up was identical (mean 24 months [range 12–36 months]).

None of the patients in this study had reactionary hemorrhage. Twenty-seven patients (5.4%) in the elective group and ten patients (4.9%) in the emergency group suffered secondary hemorrhage ($P < 0.05$). Fifteen patients (3.0%) in the elective group and 12 patients (5.9%) in the emergency group developed symptomatic anal stricture that required either anal dilatation or anoplasty ($P < 0.05$). Varying degree of fecal incontinence developed in 26 patients (5%) in the elective group, and in 9 (4%) in the emergency group ($P < 0.05$). None of the study patients developed portal pyemia or septicemia. Thirty-eight patients (7.6%) in the elective group and 14 patients (6.9%) in the emergency group developed recurrent hemorrhoids ($P < 0.05$).

We also compared stapled hemorrhoidectomy versus conventional diathermy hemorrhoidectomy for acutely thrombosed circumferentially prolapsed piles [25]. A total of 35 patients with circumferential, edematous, prolapsed piles were recruited into this trial. Eighteen patients underwent open diathermy hemorrhoidectomy, while 17 underwent stapled hemorrhoidectomy. Although patients who underwent stapled hemorrhoidectomy experienced significantly more pain at discharge, they subsequently had less pain, bleeding, and persistent symptoms requiring readmission at two weeks and at six weeks follow-up. It was thus concluded that stapled hemorrhoidectomy for acutely thrombosed circumferential piles is feasible and may result in less pain and more rapid symptom resolution compared to open hemorrhoidectomy.

The overall results for emergency hemorrhoidectomy showed no incidence of portal pyemia and a low incidence of secondary hemorrhage, stricture, or incontinence. Emergency hemorrhoidectomy offers several advantages over conservative treatment of acute hemorrhoids. Definitive hemorrhoidectomy at the time of admission saves the patient a subsequent readmission for an elective surgery. The patient is also spared the pain and discomfort of nonsurgical treatment for the acute episode, while the discomfort following emergency hemorrhoidectomy is the same as that following elective surgery. Furthermore, morbidity following emergency hemorrhoidectomy is not increased compared to that following elective hemorrhoidectomy.

Overall Results

From our latest series of 82 patients who underwent diathermy hemorrhoidectomy, three patients developed post-hemorrhoidectomy hemorrhage (3.6%). Three patients developed urinary retention (3.6%), one (1.2%) required readmission for post-hemorrhoidectomy pain. There were no patients who developed fecal incontinence or postoperative strictures. These results are comparable to if not better than the reported incidence of 0.8–4.2% of post-hemorrhoidectomy hemorrhage, 1% incidence of anal stenosis, and 0.4% incidence of incontinence in other series [26, 27, 28]. With the application of topical glyceryl trinitrate ointment, we were able to achieve complete epithelization of hemorrhoidectomy in 42.5% of patients in three weeks and 77.5% of patients by four weeks [17]. This is an improvement compared to our previous results [7].

The results of treatment of circumferential prolapsed piles by extended techniques were poorer than that of three-pile hemorrhoidectomy. Of 28 patients, one patient developed incontinence to gas and one to liquids (7.1%). Another five patients developed anal stenosis (17.8%). This is low, however, compared to complication rates of up to 34% in other series [29]. Stapled hemorrhoidectomy, however, currently offers superior results for this entity [20, 21].

Conclusion

Diathermy hemorrhoidectomy is safe, fast, and effective for the performance of open and closed hemorrhoidectomy and appropriate as well for emergency cases. Wound healing rates may be improved by topical glyceryl trinitrate which improves anodermal blood flow. The addition of methylene blue for topical analgesics may allow a prolongation of analgesic, and thus a less painful recovery.

References

1. Ho KS, Eu KW, Seow-Choen F et al. Randomized clinical trial of haemorrhoidectomy under a mixture of local anesthesia versus general anesthesia. Br J Surg 2000; 87:410–3.
2. Ho YH, Foo CL, Seow-Choen F et al. Prospective randomized controlled trial of a micronized flavonidic fraction to reduce bleeding after haemorrhoidectomy. Br J Surg 1995;38:776–7.
3. Seow-Choen F, Ho YH, Ang HG et al. Prospective, randomized trial comparing pain and clinical function after conventional scissors excision/ligation vs diathermy excision without ligation for symptomatic prolapsed haemorrhoids. Dis Colon Rectum 1992;34:1165–9.
4. Bassi R, Bergami G. The surgical treatment of haemorrhoids: diathermocoagulation and traditional technics. A prospective randomized study. Minerva Chir 1997; 52:387–91.
5. Tan JJY, Seow-Choen F. Prospective randomized trial comparing diathermy and harmonic scalpel haemorrhoidectomy. Dis Colon Rectum 2001;44:677–9.
6. Ibrahim S, Tsang C, Seow-Choen F et al. Prospective randomized trial comparing pain and clinical function between diathermy versus scissors closed haemorrhoidectomy. Dis Colon Rectum 1998;41:1418–20.
7. Ho YH, Seow-Choen F, Tan M et al. Randomized controlled trial of open and closed haemorrhoidectomy. Br J Surg 1997;84:1729–30.
8. Parks AG. The surgical treatment of haemorrhoids. Br J Surg 1956;43:337–51.
9. Roe AM, Bartolo DC, Velacott KD et al. Submucosal versus ligation haemorrhoidectomy: a comparison of anal sensation, anal sphincter manometry and postoperative pain and function. Br J Surg 1987;74:948–51.
10. Quah HM, Seow-Choen F. Prospective randomized trial comparing diathermy excision and diathermy coagulation for symptomatic prolapsed haemorrhoids. Dis Colon Rectum 2004;44:367–70.
11. Cheetham MJ, Philips RK. Evidence-based practice in haemorrhoidectomy. Colorectal Dis 2001;3:126–34.
12. Asfar SK, Juma TH, Ala-Edeen T. Hemorrhoidectomy and sphincterotomy. A prospective study comparing the effectiveness of anal stretch and sphincterotomy in reducing pain after hemorrhoidectomy. Dis Colon Rectum 1988; 31:181–5.
13. Ho YH, Seow-Choen F, Low JY et al. Randomized controlled trial of trimebutine (anal sphincter relaxant) for pain after haemorrhoidectomy. Br J Surg 1997; 84:377–379.
14. Mathai V, Ong BC, Ho YH. Randomized controlled trial of lateral sphincterotomy with haemorrhoidectomy. Br J Surg 1996;83:380–382.
15. Shouten WR, Briel JW, Auwerda JJ et al. Anal fissure: new concepts in pathogenesis and treatment. Scand J Gastroenterol Suppl 1996;218:78–81.
16. Kua KB, Kocher HM, Kelkar A et al. Effect of topical glyceryl trinitrate on anodermal blood flow in patients with chronic anal fissures. ANZ J Surg 2001;71:548–50.
17. Tan KY, Sng KK, Eu KW et al. Randomized clinical trial of 0.2 per cent glyceryl trinitrate ointment for wound healing and pain reduction after diathermy haemorrhoidectomy. Br J Surg 2006;93:1464–8.
18. Tan KY, Seow-Choen F. Methylene blue injection reduces pain after lateral anal sphincterotomy. Tech Coloproctol 2007;11:68–9.
19. Seow-Choen F, Lee HC. Prospective randomized study of radical versus four-pile haemorrhoidectomy for symptomatic large circumferential prolapsed piles. Br J Surg 1995;82:188–9.
20. Seow-Choen F. Stapled haemorrhoidectomy: pain or gain. Br J Surg 2001;88:1–3.
21. Seow-Choen F. Surgery for haemorrhoids. ablation or correction. Asian J Surg 2002;25:265–6.
22. Tinckler LF, Barathma G. Immediate haemorrhoidectomy for prolapsed piles. Lancet 1964;141:810–2.
23. Howard PM, Pingree JH. Immediate radical surgery for haemorrhoidal disease with extensive thrombosis. Am J Surg 1968;116:777–8.
24. Eu KW, Seow-Choen F, Goh HS. Comparison of emergency and elective haemorrhoidectomy. Br J Surg 1994;81:308–10.
25. Brown SR, Ballan K, Seow-Choen F et al. Stapled mucosectomy for acute thrombosed circumferentially prolapsed piles. A prospective randomized comparison with conventional haemorrhoidectomy. Colorectal Dis 2001;3:175–8.
26. Mortensen N, Romanos J. Hemorrhoids. In: Nicholls RJ, Dozois RR (eds). Surgery of the colon and rectum. 1997. Churchill Livingston, New York:224–9.
27. Johnstone CS, Ibister WH. Inpatient management of piles: a surgical audit. Aust NZ J Surg 1992;62:720–4.
28. Rosen L, Sipe P, Stasik JJ et al. Outcome of delayed hemorrhage following surgical hemorrhoidectomy. Dis Colon Rectum 1993;36:743–6.
29. Boccasanta P, Venturi M, Orio A et al. Circular hemorrhoidectomy in advanced hemorrhoidal disease. Hepatogastroenterology 1998;45:969–72.

18 Laser Hemorrhoidectomy

Edmund I. Leff

Hemorrhoidectomy has been an operation feared by patients because of the pain and occasional prolonged healing. Surgeons have turned to technology in an attempt to decrease pain, improve healing, and shorten the recovery time. Multiple in-office nonoperative procedures such as sclerotherapy, rubber band ligations, and infrared coagulation are useful for treating first-, second-, and some third-degree internal hemorrhoids. However, when there are large external hemorrhoids as well as large third- and fourth-degree hemorrhoids with or without a fissure, surgical hemorrhoidectomy remains the treatment of choice.

Lasers destroy tissue by concentrating the energy of electromagnetic radiation. The energy can be deployed diffusely over an area to ablate tissue or as a concentrated beam to cut tissue. Compared to diathermy there is less diffusion of thermal energy, which in theory causes less destruction of adjacent tissue and should promote more rapid healing. Both the Nd:Yag and CO_2 laser have been used to perform hemorrhoidectomies, and the techniques have varied greatly.

The results of performing hemorrhoidectomy with a laser have not shown consistent improvement in healing or lessening of pain. The technique used can affect the results. For instance, one surgeon doing "laser hemorrhoidectomy" rubber bands the internal hemorrhoids and destroys the tissue within the bands. This method is less painful than an operative three-quadrant hemorrhoidectomy, but is not anything more than multiple rubber band ligations in an expensive outpatient operating room. Dissecting the mucosa from the underlying sphincter with the laser rather than using scissor dissection can result in sphincter damage.

The disadvantages of using a laser are many and include:

1. The equipment, especially the Nd:Yag, is expensive and is not used in many other procedures or specialties that can defer the cost.
2. An extra circulating nurse is used in my community because of the potential fire danger, which I have experienced first hand. This raises the cost.
3. Use of the laser does not speed up the procedure, even though with some techniques pedicle ligation is not necessary.

The harmonic scalpel is another method of performing the dissection and controlling the bleeding in a hemorrhoidectomy. Advocates of this procedure claim it is less painful. In my community my colleagues and I have seen several patients with early postoperative strictures and fissures. Whether this is a consequence of the instrument or the surgeons using it is hard to assess.

In summary, the laser, whether the Nd:Yag or the CO_2, in the treatment of hemorrhoidal disease is a procedure searching for justification of the added cost. It is certainly as effective as traditional hemorrhoidectomy in skilled hands. The use of a scanner in addition to the CO_2 laser has helped in some hands. Clear and convincing evidence of less pain, better healing, and earlier return to work have not been demonstrated.

I. Khubchandani et al. (eds.), *Surgical Treatment of Hemorrhoids*, DOI 10.1007/978-1-84800-314-9_18,

References

1. Eddy HJ, Yu JC, Eddy EC. Dual laser haemorrhoidectomy [abstract] Lasers Surg Med 1986;6:201.
2. Leff EI. Haemorrhoidectomy—laser vs. non-laser: outpatient surgical experience. Dis Colon Rectum 1992;35:743–6.
3. Singapore A, Mazier PW, Luchtefeld MA et al. Treatment of advanced haemorrhoidal disease: a perspective randomized comparison of cold scalpel vs contact NdYag laser. Dis Colon Rectum 1993;36:1042–9.
4. Chungg CC, Ha JPY, Tai YP et al. Double blind, randomized trial comparing harmonic scalpel haemorrhoidectomy, bipolar scissors haemorrhoidectomy, and scissor excision: ligation technique. Dis Colon Rectum 2001;45:789–94.
5. Wang JY, Chang-Chien CR, Chien JS et al. The role of lasers in haemorrhoidectomy. Dis Colon Rectum 1991; 34:78–82.

19 Cryotherapy

John J. O'Connor

Cryotherapy is not new. It enjoyed an early enthusiasm in the 1970s for the treatment of anorectal disease, particularly hemorrhoids. It represented an attempt to replace standard surgical excision of hemorrhoids by a less invasive, less painful, and less expensive method. This search still continues today with the infrared photocoagulator, multiple bandings, and, more recently, the procedure for prolapsing hemorrhoids (stapled hemorrhoidectomy).

A web search still provides information regarding cryohemorrhoidectomy. The website of the American Society of Colon and Rectal Surgeons states: "Cryotherapy is an effective alternative with the least side effects when directed at first degree and second degree hemorrhoids. It is not recommended for use with external hemorrhoids. Some physicians treat third degree hemorrhoids with cryotherapy" [1]. The 1st European Congress on Cryosurgery in 2000 reported: "It is used as a curative treatment in villous tumors, condyloma, fistula, pilonidal cysts, hemorrhoids, and it offers a minimally invasive procedure, very well tolerated, and very effective and cost-effective treatment [2]." A further search of the web lists a health site discussing cryotherapy for hemorrhoids. Pillwatch.com lists cryotherapy as a nonsurgical alternative [3]. The Broward County Medical Examiner's Office website also lists cryotherapy as an alternative to surgery [4].

It is safe to say that there seems to be little support for cryotherapy in the United States. Few surgeons today employ this method. Mann correctly devotes little space to this in the 2002 edition of his textbook [5]. Cryosurgery can be used for second-degree internal hemorrhoids, but bleeding is a greater problem when it is used than if ligation or infrared photocoagulation is used. The procedure is also more cumbersome, takes longer, and does cause pain. It should be noted that the current clinic in colon and rectal surgery under the section of hemorrhoids does not even mention cryosurgery as an alternative.

As one who was active in the development of cryohemorrhoidectomy, I now believe better methods have been developed. I feel cryohemorrhoidectomy belongs in the class of "nothing ventured nothing gained," and I can no longer recommend or advise cryotherapy for the treatment of internal hemorrhoids.

References

1. American Society of Colon and Rectal Surgeons. Revised 2003 website.
2. 1st European Congress on Cryosurgery—Donostia-San Sebastian, Spain, April 2000.
3. Pillwatch.com.
4. Broward County Florida Office Medical Examiner Website.
5. Mann CV. Surgical treatment of haemorrhoids. 2002: 129–131. Springer-Verlag, London

I. Khubchandani et al. (eds.), *Surgical Treatment of Hemorrhoids*, DOI 10.1007/978-1-84800-314-9_19,
© Springer-Verlag London Limited 2009

20 Complications of Surgical Hemorrhoidectomy

Salim Amrani and Marvin L. Corman

A number of treatment modalities are available for the management of hemorrhoids, including a host of office procedures as well as surgery. In recent years most of the surgical literature has focused on the so-called stapled hemorrhoidopexy. This chapter addresses the complications of surgical hemorrhoidectomy and those of stapled hemorrhoidopexy.

The following is a partial list of the potential problems of surgical hemorrhoidectomy:

- Pain
- Urinary retention
- Urinary tract infection
- Constipation
- Fecal impaction
- hemorrhage
- Infection
- Anal tags
- Mucosal prolapse
- Mucosal ectropion
- Rectal stricture
- Anal fissure

Pain

Although pain is not actually a complication of surgery, it is nonetheless the single most important reason why patients avoid hemorrhoidectomy. The etiology of pain after hemorrhoidectomy is multifactorial—the trauma caused by the incision to the sensitive anoderm, internal sphincter spasm, and inflammation consequent to the incisions. A

number of diverse methods of treatment for this pervasive concern have been described.

The reality is that with the preference, if not the requirement, for outpatient surgery, one cannot rely on the full armamentarium of approaches to deal with pain (e.g., patient-controlled analgesia and epidural morphine) [1].

Goldstein and colleagues suggest a subcutaneous morphine pump for postoperative pain management [2]. Although theirs was not a controlled study, the authors concluded that the combination of outpatient hemorrhoidectomy and the pump was cost-effective when compared to inpatient management.

Toradol® (ketorolac tromethamine) has also been advocated as uniquely beneficial for anorectal surgery. Generally, 60 mg (2 ml) is injected directly into the anal sphincter at the time of its exposure during hemorrhoidectomy. Studies suggest that there is a much reduced level not only of pain, but also of the incidence of urinary retention [3, 4].

Flagyl® (metronidazole) in its oral form has been recommended as an effective medication for ameliorating pain following hemorrhoidectomy, but in a randomized, double-blind trial, Balfour and coworkers failed to support this conclusion [5]. Additionally, topical metronidazole (10%) used in a prospective, randomized trial showed reduction of pain at postoperative days 7 and 14 compared with placebo [6].

Different strategies have been used to decrease the sphincter spasm that has been felt to

I. Khubchandani et al. (eds.), *Surgical Treatment of Hemorrhoids*, DOI 10.1007/978-1-84800-314-9_20,
© Springer-Verlag London Limited 2009

contribute to the pain. Nitroglycerin ointment (0.2%) and Nitroderm TTS band application have demonstrated reduction of pain in randomized trials [7, 8]. Headaches however, are a real problem.

Davies and colleagues undertook a double-blind study of 50 consecutive patients who underwent Milligan-Morgan hemorrhoidectomy and randomly assigned an internal sphincter injection of 0.4 ml of a solution containing either botulinum toxin (20 U: Botox) or normal saline [9]. Those who received the toxin injection had a significant pain reduction at days 6 and 7. Patti and colleagues showed significant reduction in pain and time of healing, and earlier return to work in a group of patients receiving botulinum toxin injection compared with normal saline in a randomized control trial, with a correlation between the amount of pain and the measured maximum postoperative resting pressure [10].

Internal anal sphincterotomy and sphincter stretch are not recommended to ameliorate pain, since they are not effective and risk some level of impairment for bowel control [11].

Urinary Retention

Urinary retention is the most common complication following hemorrhoidectomy. Bleday and coworkers reported a 20% incidence [12]. Factors often held responsible include the following:

- Spinal anesthesia
- Rectal pain and spasm
- High ligation of the hemorrhoidal pedicle
- Rough handling of tissue
- Heavy suture material
- Numerous sutures
- Fluid overload
- Tight, bulky dressings
- Anti-cholinergics
- Narcotics [13, 14, 15, 16]

Pain and fluid overload are the primary factors that contribute to urinary retention [17, 18]. If pain medication is inadequate, the patient cannot relax the sphincter mechanism sufficiently to urinate. It simply hurts too much, on top of which the pain inhibits the detrusor muscle, causing the bladder to fail to empty. One must limit fluids; this requires education of the anesthesiologist, the nurses, and house officers. Frightening the patient with a catheter or leaving standing orders for catheterization is a self-fulfilling prophecy for its subsequent insertion. The patient should void before the operation, the minimal intravenous infusion necessary is given during the procedure [19], and the infusion is terminated in the recovery room. Bladder distention is deleterious for detrusor contractility [19]. If hospital regulations require that an intravenous line be maintained, a heparin lock will suffice.

Oral fluids are restricted until the following morning. Finally, patients are not routinely catheterized; this is carried out only when the bladder is distended or the patient complains, and then only after examination by a physician [20]. In the morning, with the commencement of sitz baths, most patients will void who have not already done so. Once the nursing service has been educated not even to inquire about voiding, the incidence of retention and the associated complication of urinary tract infection will be significantly reduced. Pudendal nerve block has been shown to be superior to spinal anesthesia with regard to voiding complications. By this technique Kim and colleagues reduced the incidence of catheterization from 69.6% to 7.5% [21].

If a urinary catheter is placed, it should remain for 24 h if the residual urine is more than 500 ml, because it is unlikely that the patient will be able to void subsequently. Conversely, with a residual of less than 500 ml, the catheter can be removed with a reasonable expectation that spontaneous urination will occur. It is possible through the use of portable ultrasound technology to measure bladder volume and to avoid unnecessary catheterization. Pavlin and coworkers, using a Bladder Manager® PCI 5000 (Diagnostic Ultrasound, Redmond, WA), studied outpatient surgery individuals and concluded that bladder monitoring in high-risk patients for urinary retention (including anal surgery), facilitated deciding when a patient should be catheterized [22].

Urinary Tract Infection

Urinary tract infection is usually a direct consequence of catheterization for urinary retention. The most common offending organisms are coliform bacteria. Appropriate antibiotics and catheter removal usually result in rapid resolution, but chronic infection, cystitis, and pyelonephritis can be late sequelae. Here again, the value of avoiding urinary retention cannot be overestimated.

Constipation

Patients who undergo hemorrhoidectomy await their postoperative bowel evacuation less than enthusiastically and often view the enema intended to facilitate this function with apprehension. The consequence of untreated constipation will likely lead to fecal impaction which will in turn further complicate management. The pain managed by the generous administration of narcotics plays an important role in the etiology of constipation. Opiate analgesics act centrally to control pain, but also peripherally to promote constipation by slowing intestinal transit and by limiting water secretion. This effect is caused by direct action on the enteric nervous system through μ-opioid receptors [23]. The effect of general anesthesia, local physiologic dysfunction resulting from surgical manipulation, and lack of ambulation all contribute to constipation [24]. A history of irregular bowel function and colonic hypomotility may complicate the problem further.

Constipation should, of course, be prevented. Instructions to the patient should include a discussion on bowel management. A high-fiber diet is recommended. Ample water intake should be started as soon as the patient can urinate, bulking agents and laxatives prescribed, and ambulation encouraged [25]. We recommend a stimulant laxative to be started on the evening of the operation and continued in increasing doses until defecation occurs [26]. Non-opioid analgesics should be prescribed concomitantly with opioids to limit the requirement for constipating medications. New medications are being developed to antagonize the opioid gastrointestinal effect, such as the addition of a μ-opioid receptor antagonist [27, 28].

One should expect to defecate by the second or third postoperative day. By the third postoperative day with no bowel action, a vigorous laxative, such as Fleet phospho-soda or magnesium citrate, should be considered. If no bowel movement occurs by the fourth day, a gentle enema may be administered.

Hemorrhage

Hemorrhage after hemorrhoidectomy is relatively rare (0.6–5.4%) and can be early or delayed [29]. Failure to adequately ligate the hemorrhoid pedicle is the cause of bleeding within the first 24 h; therefore, the pedicle should be suture-ligated and not simply hand-tied. If this complication develops, the patient requires emergency intervention. Proposed temporizing methods include direct pressure application with a finger or gauze and submucosal injection of 1–2 ml of 1:100,000 epinephrine. Packing is to be condemned. Suture ligation of the bleeding pedicle in the operating room is the most effective, most reassuring, and the safest alternative [30].

Delayed hemorrhage is a complication of both the open and the closed hemorrhoidectomy and occurs usually 7–14 days postoperatively. It is believed to be due to sepsis in the pedicle or erosion of the suture, although some authors do not support this concept [29]. Chen and colleagues presented a series of 4,880 consecutive hemorrhoidectomies and suggested that male gender and a surgeon's inexperience are independent risk factors contributing to posthemorrhoidectomy hemorrhage [29]. They observed that none of the bleeding patients in their series had pyrexia, signs of sepsis, or wound infection. They concluded that surgeons with more experience and seniority had a lower incidence of hemorrhage, implying that the incidence of delayed hemorrhage is related to the technical ability of the surgeon.

Delayed bleeding warrants an examination, including anoscopy. Treatment may vary from expectant management with in-hospital observation alone. Alternatively, bedside anal packing using a rolled, slightly moistened gelatin sponge (Gelfoam) [31], transfusion, and resuturing may be required. Some have employed a Foley catheter technique for tamponading the bleeding point, with reported success in all five individuals so treated [32].

Local Infection and Sepsis

It seems counterintuitive that since hemorrhoidectomy is carried out in a field with numerous and varied bacterial organisms present, there is not a higher incidence of septic complications following this operation. However, it is important to be wary of immunocompromised patients and those with valvular heart disease. Antibiotic prophylaxis is recommended in these individuals. Lal and Levitan have pointed out that hemomorrhoidectomy may be followed by transient bacteremia and a low-grade fever as a consequence of the relatively continuous release of bacteria into the blood stream from the maneuvering [33]. For example, an 8.5% rate of bacteremia has been reported following proctoscopic examination of patients with no evidence of lower intestinal disease [34].

It has been hypothesized that the major venous drainage of the rectum, by passing through the superior hemorhoidal veins into the portal system, clears organisms through the reticuloendothelial system of the liver. This is thought to account for explaining the low infectious complication rate following hemorrhoidectomy. The anal wounds following hemorrhoidectomy are colonized by lower gastrointestinal tract bacteria as well as by skin bacteria without overt wound infection [35]. Sitz baths, being routine in the postoperative management, may theoretically prevent most skin problems (e.g., cellulitis and

abscess). In an experience of well over 1,000 hemorrhoidectomies, one of us (MLC) cannot recall ever having to drain an abscess in the postoperative period. Fournier's gangrene has been a reported complication of this operation in both immunocompromised and non-immunocompromised patients. This rare problem is unpredictable and cannot be attributed to a particular technique [36, 37].

Anal Tags

Anal tags, which can interfere with proper cleansing of the anus and lead to skin irritation, can usually be avoided by excising the redundant skin at the time of operation. We suspect, however, that tags more often than not are the result of the manner in which the wounds heal, perhaps analogous to keloid formation in other incision sites. Bothersome tags can be excised as an office procedure if symptoms warrant.

Mucosal Prolapse

Inadequate removal of redundant, mobile rectal mucosa at the time of hemmorhoidectomy may result in mucosal prolapse. Patients may complain of a lump that requires manual reduction. Problems with mucous discharge and pruritic symptoms are common. Treatment usually consists of rubber ring ligation of the prolapsed mucosa. If there seems to be extensive or circumferential involvement, the surgeon should conduct the examination while the patient strains on the toilet, in order to look for procidentia. Prevention of this complication requires that the surgeon remove any redundant mucosa at the time of hemorrhoidectomy. It will be interesting to note whether there is an increased incidence of recurrent prolapse following stapled hemorrhoidopexy.

Ectropion

Ectropion is also called wet anus or Whitehead deformity. This complication occurs because the redundant rectal mucosa has a tendency to descend and even to heal outside the anal verge. The surgeon should anchor the mucosa to the underlying internal sphincter if redundant mucosa is noted. If the surgeon anchors the mucosa to the skin in one or more quadrants, a partial ectropion may result. Interestingly, Khubchandani has reported treatment of anal stenosis by doing just what has been condemned, that is, advancing the mucosa, albeit not beyond the anal verge [38]. Ectropion can lead to mucous discharge, skin irritation, and pruritus ani. As long as no stricture is present, simple excision and transverse suture of the wound edge to the underlying internal anal sphincter will suffice. The open wound should heal without the mucosal extrusion. An alternative approach is to perform an anoplasty.

Anal Stricture

This condition is a consequence of replacement of normal tissue with fibrous scar. This may develop following extensive removal of encircling hemorrhoids, thereby leading to contraction of the anorectal outlet. When healing is complete, a narrow, foreshortened, stenotic orifice may remain.

This is a preventable complication, especially if the surgeon makes every possible effort to preserve skin bridges. However, in the presence of gangrenous hemorrhoids, distortion of the anal canal, chronic fibrosis, chronic fissure, external tags, and hypertrophied anal papillae, extensive removal of involved tissue is often necessary to accomplish an adequate hemorrhoidectomy. Under these circumstances the surgeon can either compromise on the amount of tissue removed and accept the consequences of patient complaints of residual disease, or consider the possibility of performing an anoplasty at the time of hemorrhoidectomy.

Treatment includes laxatives, suppositories, dilation, enemas, or surgical intervention. This last treatment may consist of excision of eschar and sphincterotomy, but for a more profound stenosis a formal anoplasty should be performed. This may involve one of a number of types of advancement flaps, rotation flaps, or pedicle flaps.

Rectal Stricture

Stricture of the rectum is a rare sequela of hemorrhoidectomy and usually is misdiagnosed as an *anal* stricture. The complication is caused by vigorous high ligation of the hemorrhoid pedicles that strips the rectal mucosa in several areas. It is most likely to occur if the patient has an element of prolapse or laxity of the rectal mucosa. As with virtually all complications, prevention is the best approach. Care must be taken to avoid gathering a mass of rectal lining into the ligatures. Management of this complication may require dilation, either with Young's dilators if the stricture is distal, or a Hegar dilator if the stricture is higher. Operative lysis may be necessary, possibly including either advancement of the rectal mucosa or proctoplasty.

Fissure or Ulcer

An anal fissure may develop in a patient who has a contracted anorectal outlet after hemorrhoidectomy. Usually, the fissure is situated posteriorly. Repeated trauma from defecation results in laceration of the eschar, which may become a chronic painful anal ulcer. Such postoperative fissures may respond to conservative management (e.g., laxatives, enemas, suppositories, topical creams such as cortisone) and dilation. However, often an additional procedure is required, most commonly an internal anal sphincterotomy. Excision of the ulcer concomitant with the sphincterotomy may be of benefit, but some form of anoplasty may ultimately be required to increase anal canal circumference.

Pseudopolyps

Hemorrhoidectomy usually requires ligation of the stump of the hemorrhoid. Tissue strangulation may take place at the site of ligation, resulting in sloughing of the stump. This leaves a defect that heals by granulation, the end result of which may be a pseudopolyp. Another possible contributing factor is a foreign-body granuloma, which may be a consequence of the prolonged presence of suture material [39]. This may be manifested by an edematous, polypoid, or sessile tumor at the site of the suture. Pseudopolyps can be excised with a local anesthetic or be electrocoagulated.

Epidermal Cyst

In rare instances, some months after hemorrhoidectomy, asymptomatic inclusion cysts may appear in the anal canal or in the immediate perianal region. Their origin has been attributed to retention of keratin elements, hair particles, or exfoliated squamous epithelial cells in the wound. If these cysts are bothersome, they can be removed by local excision.

Anal Fistula

Anal fistula is an unusual complication of hemorrhoidectomy, occurring in approximately 1% of patients. It is allegedly more common after the closed operation than the open, but the incidence is so low that this observation is probably more theoretical than factual. The fistula is inevitably low and subcutaneous, not transsphincteric or even intersphincteric, unless the finding is coincidental. Fistulotomy is the appropriate treatment and can often be accomplished in the office.

Pruritus Ani

Most causes of pruritus ani are related to diet or are caused by overaggressive attention to anal hygiene. However, pruritic symptoms following hemorrhoidectomy are not unusual and may actually have an anatomic basis. A mucosal ectropion or Whitehead deformity, for example, can produce mucous discharge, which can contribute to the pruritus. With a specific anatomic abnormality, anoplasty may be advisable.

Fecal Incontinence

Fecal soilage or incontinence following hemorrhoidectomy, although infrequent, is not as rare as the physician might expect. A possible explanation is the loss of anal canal sensation resulting from removal of sensory-bearing tissue and its replacement by scar. We do not subscribe to such a theory.

Almost all patients who have impairment of fecal control following hemorrhoidectomy are elderly. If the physician takes a careful history, it will probably be discovered that many of these individuals have experienced soilage before the operation, although the procedure may have exacerbated the problem. This is often the case when the patient has some degree of mucosal or rectal prolapse, and it is a particular concern in women. Special care should be taken when performing this operation in the older age group.

It is important to avoid unnecessary sphincter stretch or sphincterotomy. Many surgeons are fond of sphincterotomy, because they believe it ameliorates the postoperative pain problem. This has not been found to be true when studied in trials. When it is performed at the posterior pile site, a keyhole deformity can result. It is a potentially hazardous maneuver in an individual without a concomitant fissure and should be avoided, especially in someone older than 60 years of age.

Recurrence

Most patients who complain of recurrent hemorrhoids usually are describing skin tags or have pruritic symptoms. However, in some cases, true hemorrhoidal veins have developed that have become symptomatic after an assumed complete hemorrhoidectomy. "Doctor, I had the operation 10 years ago, and now the hemorrhoids are back," is the expressed observation. However, piles that have been removed cannot recur. The "recurrence" consists of veins that, either because of their normal appearance at the time of hemorrhoidectomy or in an effort to preserve adequate mucosal bridges, were left undisturbed. With increased pressure or collateral circulation developing over the years, dilatation occurs and symptomatic hemorrhoids may result.

Because of this potential problem, all hemorrhoidal veins should be removed at the time of the surgical procedure. Tunneling out minute vessels from the underlying mucosa and debriding all veins over the external sphincter are important prophylactic maneuvers. When recurrent piles become symptomatic, ideal treatment should be by an outpatient procedure, usually rubber band ligation or office excision.

Retroperitoneal Air

A solitary case of retroperitoneal air following hemorrhoidectomy was reported by Kriss and colleagues [40]. The patient had been receiving steroids for rheumatoid arthritis, so this medication may have played some part in its occurrence. The authors suggested that air was introduced either during the dissection or subsequently, when the patient coughed or strained. The patient responded well to nonoperative management.

Complications of Stapled Hemorrhoidopexy

While stapled hemorrhoidopexy is thought to be as effective as conventional hemorrhoidectomy, with the advantages of less pain and earlier return to work [41, 42, 43, 44, 45], disconcerting complications have been described since the introduction of this technique in 1998. These consist mainly of an increased risk of septic complications from rectal perforation, such as pelvic abscess and retroperitoneal sepsis [46, 47, 48, 49]. Rectovaginal fistula is a unique complication from this operation, presumably occurring if the vagina is incorporated in the circular stapled closure. Pescatori and coworkers describe a rectal pocket syndrome [50]. This is characterized by the formation of a deep cavity, resembling a wide intramural sinus, with an internal orifice communicating with the rectal lumen at the level of the staple line. This can harbor fecal matter and be the source of local sepsis, irritation, and pain. The treatment proposed by the authors is to lay open and curette the cavity [50].

This operation has similar complications to that of conventional surgical hemorrhoidectomy, including pain, urinary retention, bleeding, anal stenosis, anal incontinence, and granuloma formation. With respect to pain, some have attributed this to staples having been deployed too low (i.e., within the anal canal), but persistent pain may occur for many months despite observation of what appears to be an ideal staple line level.

References

1. Kuo R-J. Epidural morphine for posthemorrhoidectomy analgesia. Dis Colon Rectum 1984;27:529–30.
2. Goldstein ET, Williamson PR, Larach SW. Subcutaneous morphine pump for postoperative hemorrhoidectomy pain management. Dis Colon Rectum 1993;36:439–46.
3. O'Donovan S, Ferrara A, Larach S et al. Intraoperative use of Toradol facilitates outpatient hemorrhoidectomy. Dis Colon Rectun 1994;37:793–9.
4. Richman IM. Use of Toradol in anorectal surgery. Dis Colon Rectum 1993;36:295–6.

5. Balfour L, Stojkovic SG, Botterill ID et al. A randomized, double-blind trial of the effect of metronidazole on pain after closed hemorrhoidectomy. Dis Colon Rectum 2002; 45:1186–90.

6. Nicholson TJ, Armstrong D. Topical metronidazole (10%) decreases posthemorrhoidectomy pain and improves healing. Dis Colon Rectum 2004;47:711–6.

7. Coskun A, Duzgun SA, Uzunkoy A et al. Nitroderm TTS band application for pain after hemorrhoidectomy. Dis Colon Rectum 2001;44:680–5.

8. Wasvary HJ, Hain J, Mosed-Vogel M et al. Randomized, prospective, double-blind, placebo-controlled trial of effect of nitroglycerine ointment on pain after hemorrhoidectomy. Dis Colon Rectum 2001;44:1069–73.

9. Davies J, Duffy D, Boyt N et al. Botulinum toxin (Botox®) reduces pain after hemorrhoidectomy: results of a double-blind, randomized study. Dis Colon Rectum 2003; 46:1097–102.

10. Patti R, Almasio PL, Muggeo VMR et al. Improvement of wound healing after hemorrhoidectomy: a double-blind, randomized study of botulinum toxin injection. Dis Colon Rectum 2005;48:2173–9.

11. Khubchandani IT. Internal sphincterotomy with hemorrhoidectomy does not relieve pain: a prospective, randomized study. Dis Colon Rectum 2002;45:1452–7.

12. Bleday R, Pena JP, Rothenberger DA et al. Symptomatic hemorrhoids: current incidence and complications of operative therapy. Dis Colon Rectum 1992;35:477–81.

13. Crystal RF, Hopping RA. Early postoperative complications of anorectal surgery. Dis Colon Rectum 1974; 17:336–41.

14. Kratzer GL. Local anesthesia in anorectal surgery. Dis Colon Rectum 1965;8:441–5.

15. Nesselrod JP. Clinical proctology, 3rd ed. Philadelphia: WB Saunders, 1964.

16. Salvati EP. Urinary retention in anorectal and colonic surgery. Am J Surg 1957;94:114–7.

17. Bailey HR, Ferguson JA. Prevention of urinary retention by fluid restriction following anorectal operations. Dis Colon Rectum 1976;19:250–2.

18. Scoma JA. Hemorrhoidectomy without urinary retention and catheterization. Conn Med 1976;40:751–2.

19. Petros, JG, Bradley, TM. Factors influencing postoperative urinary retention in patients undergoing surgery for benign anorectal disease. Am J Surg 1990;159:374–6.

20. Tammela T, Kontturi M, Lukkarinen O. Postoperative urinary retention: incidence and predisposing factors. Scand J Urol Nephrol 1986;20:197–201.

21. Kim J, Lee DS, Jang SM et al. The effect of pudendal block on voiding after hemorrhoidectomy. Dis Colon Rectum 2005;48:518–23.

22. Pavlin DJ, Pavlin EG, Gunn HC et al. Voiding in patients managed with or without ultrasound monitoring of bladder volume after outpatient surgery. Anesth Analg 1999; 89:90–7.

23. Bohn LM, Raehal K. Opioid receptor signaling: relevance for gastrointestinal therapy. Curr Opin Pharmacol 2006; 6:559–63.

24. Stevens RA, Mikat-Stevens M, Flanigan R et al. Does the choice of anesthetic technique affect the recovery of bowel function after radical prostatectomy? Urology 1998; 52:213–8.

25. Johnson CD, Budd J, Ward AJ. Laxatives after hemorrhoidectomy. Dis Colon Rectum 1987;30:780–1.

26. Corman ML. Management of postoperative constipation in anorectal surgery. Dis Colon Rectum 1979;22:149–51.

27. Delaney CP, Weese JL, Hyman NH et al. Phase III trial of alvimopan, a novel, peripherally acting, mu-opioid antagonist, for postoperative ileus after major abdominal surgery. Dis Colon Rectum 2005;48:1114–25.

28. Holzer P. Treatment of opioid-induced gut dysfunction. Expert Opin Investig Drugs 2007;16:181–94.

29. Chen HH, Wang JY, Changchien CR. Risk factors associated with posthemorrhoidectomy secondary hemorrhage. Dis Colon Rectum 2002;45:1096–9.

30. Nyam DC, Seow-Choen F, Ho YH. Submucosal adrenaline injection for posthemorrhoidectomy hemorrhage. Dis Colon Rectum 1995;38:776–7.

31. Rosen L, Sipe P, Stasik JJ et al. Outcome of delayed hemorrhage following surgical hemorrhoidectomy. Dis Colon Rectum 1993;36:743–6.

32. Basso L, Pescatori M. Outcome of delayed hemorrhage following surgical hemorrhoidectomy [Letter]. Dis Colon Rectum 1994;37:288–9.

33. Lal D, Levitan R. Bacteremia following proctoscopic biopsy of a rectal polyp. Arch Intern Med 1972;130:127–8.

34. LeFrock JL, Ellis CA, Turchik JB et al. Transient bacteremia associated with sigmoidoscopy. N Engl J Med 1973;289:467–9.

35. DePaula PR, Speranzini MB, Hamzagic HC et al. Bacteriology of the anal wound after open hemorrhoidectomy: qualitative and quantitative analysis. Dis Colon Rectum 1991;34:664–9.

36. Lenhardt M, Steinstraesser L, Druecke D et al. Fournier's gangrene after Milligan-Morgan hemorrhoidectomy requiring subsequent abdominoperineal resection of the rectum: report of a case. Dis Colon Rectum 2004; 47:1729–33.

37. Cihan A, Mentes BB, Sucak G et al. Fournier's gangrene after hemorrhoidectomy: association with drug-induced agranulocytosis. Dis Colon Rectum 1999;42:1944–8.

38. Khubchandani IT. Mucosal advancement anoplasty. Dis Colon Rectum 1985;28:194–6.

39. Gaskin ER, Childers MD Jr. Increased granuloma formation from absorbable sutures. JAMA 1963;185:212–4.

40. Kriss BD, Porter JA, Slezak FA. Retroperitoneal air after routine hemorrhoidectomy: report of a case. Dis Colon Rectum 1990;33:971–3.

41. Correa-Rovelo JM, Tellez O, Obregon L et al. Stapled rectal mucosectomy vs. closed hemorrhoidectomy: a randomized clinical trial. Dis Colon Rectum 2002;45:1367–74.

42. Ganio E, Altomare DF, Gabrielli F et al. Prospective randomized multicenter trial comparing stapled with open haemorrhoidectomy. Br J Surj 2001;88:669–74.

43. Rowsell M, Bello M, Hemingway DM. Circumferential mucosectomy (stapled hemorrhoidectomy) versus conventional haemorrhoidectomy: randomized controlled trial. Lancet 2000;355:779–81.

44. Singer MA, Cintron JR, Fleshman JW et al. Early experience with stapled hemorrhoidectomy in the United States. Dis Colon Rectum 2002;45:360–7.

45. Senagore AJ, Singer M, Abcarian A et al. A prospective, randomized, controlled multicenter trial comparing stapled hemorrhoidopexy and Ferguson hemorrhoidectomy: perioperative and one-year results. Dis Colon Rectum 2004;47:1824–36.

46. Molloy R, Kingsmore D. Life-threatening pelvic sepsis after stapled haemorrhoidectomy. Lancet 2000;355:810.

47. Herold A, Kirsch J, Staude G et al. A German multicenter study on circular stapled haemorrhoidectomy. Colorectal Dis 2000;2(suppl):18.
48. Maw A, Eu K, Seow-Choen F. Retroperitoneal sepsis complicating stapled hemorrhoidectomy. Dis Colon Rectum 2002;45:826–8.
49. Wong L, Jiang J, Chang S et al. Rectal perforation: a life-threatening complication of stapled hemorrhoidectomy. Dis Colon Rectum 2003;46:116–7.
50. Pescatori M, Spyrou M, Cobellis L et al. The rectal pocket syndrome after stapled mucosectomy. Colorectal Dis 2006;8:808–11.

21 Management of Hemorrhoid Complications: Thrombosis, Fissure-in-Ano

Nina J. Paonessa

Thrombosed External Hemorrhoids

External hemorrhoids are located below the dentate line and are covered by anoderm. The typical presentation of a thrombosed external hemorrhoid is that of acute onset of perianal pain and an associated perianal lump. The pain peaks within 48 hours and usually diminishes after the fourth day [1]. Patients usually report an episode of straining, exertion (heavy lifting, exercise), or a long bicycle, car, or plane ride (i.e., prolonged sitting). If no treatment is administered, the thrombus will either spontaneously drain through the overlying skin or will reabsorb in two to four weeks [2]. What remains is an anal skin tag.

Treatment is directed toward the patient's symptoms. If the patient presents early, in acute pain, the treatment of choice is local excision [1, 2, 3]. This is performed with local anesthetic (0.5% lidocaine/0.5% Marcaine with 1:200,000 epinephrine). The patient is placed in the prone jackknife or lateral recumbent position. An elliptical incision is made over the thrombus and the overlying skin and thrombus are excised. Often the thrombus is multiloculated and therefore all clot must be removed. The skin may be left open or closed with absorbable suture (i.e., 5.0 Dexon). We choose to leave the skin open because there is less postoperative pain. The patient is instructed to use sitz baths one to two times a day and after each bowel movement. Nonsteroidal anti-inflammatory agents are all that is usually needed for incisional discomfort.

If the patient presents later in the course and is not in acute pain, conservative measures are recommended. This is in the form of sitz baths, stool-bulking agents and pain medication. Once the patient is more comfortable, anoscopic and proctoscopic examinations should be performed to assess for any anorectal disease.

Thrombosed Internal Hemorrhoids (Strangulated Hemorrhoids)

The patient that presents with strangulated internal hemorrhoids is usually in acute distress. Most have a difficult time sitting and perhaps even walking or standing, secondary to the extreme discomfort. Some patients may also have urinary retention. Strangulated hemorrhoids are the result of third- and fourth-degree hemorrhoids that have prolapsed and become irreducible secondary to swelling. Often times the edema progresses to ulceration and necrosis (see Fig. 21.1).

The treatment for strangulated internal hemorrhoids is urgent or emergent hemorrhoidectomy [1, 2]. This can be performed in the

I. Khubchandani et al. (eds.), *Surgical Treatment of Hemorrhoids*, DOI 10.1007/978-1-84800-314-9_21,
© Springer-Verlag London Limited 2009

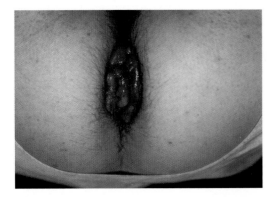

Figure 21.1 Strangulated, thrombosed internal hemorrhoids

outpatient setting. A closed hemorrhoidectomy as described in Chapter 12 is the preferred technique. An antibiotic is not indicated [1]. If more than one quadrant is excised, care must be taken to maintain at least a one-centimeter bridge of mucosa and anoderm between excision sites. All necrotic tissue should be excised [1, 4, 5, 6]. Postoperative recovery should be similar to that of patients undergoing elective hemorrhoidectomy [2].

Conservative, nonoperative management of strangulated hemorrhoids has also been described. This may be the safer option for those surgeons who are not experienced in performing a hemorrhoidectomy in complicated situations such as strangulation, where the normal anatomy is distorted. Conservative management involves relieving the pain with analgesics (intravenous if necessary); reducing perianal swelling with either hot soaks, sitz baths, or ice packs; bed rest; and prevention of constipation [3].

Fissure-in-Ano

Hemorrhoids are often associated with a fissure-in-ano. Treatment is centered on the chief complaint. If a patient has the typical symptoms of a fissure-in-ano (i.e., pain and bleeding with a bowel movement) and only first- or second-degree hemorrhoids, the fissure should be treated as the primary disease. This may be initiated with medical management. Once the fissure heals, the hemorrhoids can be treated however the surgeon deems appropriate.

The patient that presents with a nonhealing fissure, or prolapsed hemorrhoids and a symptomatic fissure, may undergo hemorrhoidectomy in conjunction with a partial sphincterotomy. The sphincterotomy may be performed at the site of the hemorrhoidectomy in most cases.

References

1. Nivatvongs S. Hemorrhoids. In: Gordon PH, Nivatvongs S. Principles and practice of surgery for the colon, rectum and anus, 2nd ed. Quality Medical Publishing, Inc. 2007:144–166.
2. Beck DE. Hemorrhoidal disease. In: Beck DE, Wexner SD. Fundamentals of anorectal surgery, 2nd ed. Elsevier Science Limited, 2002:237–253.
3. Mann CE. Management of hemorrhoid complications. In: Mann CE (ed). Surgical treatment of haemorrhoids. Springer-Verlag, London, 2002:145–153.
4. Eu KW, Seow-Cheon F, Goh HS. Comparison of emergency and elective hemorrhoidectomy. Br J Surg 1994;81:308–310.
5. Sacco S, Mortilla MG, Tonielli E, Morganti I, Cola B. Emergency hemorrhoidectomy for complicated hemorrhoids. Coloproctology 1987;9:157–159.
6. Allen PIM, Goldman M. Prolapsed thrombosed piles: a reappraisal. Coloproctology 1987;9:210–212.

22 Treatment of Hemorrhoids Complicated by Comorbidity

Nina J. Paonessa

Introduction

Hemorrhoidal symptoms are very common and may affect patients of any age or with varied comorbidities. Depending upon the severity of the comorbidity, treatment of hemorrhoids may be complicated and may require a multidisciplinary approach. It is important to remember that the goal of hemorrhoidal treatment is not to compromise the status of the patient with comorbidities.

Hemorrhoids with Inflammatory Bowel Disease

Ulcerative Colitis

Hemorrhoidal disease is not very common in patients with inflammatory bowel disease (IBD). However, similar symptoms of perianal itching, burning, and swelling from the diarrhea of IBD is common. As such, it is important to distinguish between the two disease entities when evaluating each patient. In one of the few studies describing hemorrhoids and IBD, of 50,000 patients treated at St. Mark's Hospital from 1935 to 1975, only 66 patients had IBD [1]. This same study reported a local complication rate of 7% in treating patients with ulcerative colitis and hemorrhoidectomy. It was suggested to use less invasive approaches such as injection sclerotherapy and rubber band ligation where applicable and to reserve hemorrhoidectomy for large hemorrhoids. In those patients who may have the potential to undergo a total proctocolectomy and ileal pouch reconstruction in the future, hemorrhoidectomy should be avoided because it reduces anal canal sensation.

Crohn's Disease

Again, it is very common for patients with IBD to experience perianal symptoms of itching, burning, and swelling secondary to diarrhea and not from hemorrhoids. This is especially true of the 25% of Crohn's patients with small bowel disease and perianal involvement. Another 47–50% of patients with Crohn's colitis will have anal involvement as well [2, 3]. As such, it is very important to distinguish Crohn's symptoms from hemorrhoidal symptoms. It is very well known that if the Crohn's disease in the proximal bowel, whether small bowel or colon, is not treated and under control, the perianal symptoms will not improve.

In the study from St. Mark's mentioned above, the complication rate from hemorrhoidectomy in Crohn's patients was very high (42%), and more often led to proctectomy [1]. In a more recent retrospective study performed by Wolkomir et al. in 1993, the results of hemorrhoidectomy in Crohn's patients were much more favorable. They found that in 17 patients with known

I. Khubchandani et al. (eds.), *Surgical Treatment of Hemorrhoids*, DOI 10.1007/978-1-84800-314-9_22,
© Springer-Verlag London Limited 2009

Crohn's disease in the quiescent state, 15 of the wounds healed without complications. No patient required proctectomy as a result of the hemorrhoidectomy [4].

Immunosuppression

Management of hemorrhoidal disease in the immunocompromised patient should be approached very cautiously and conservatively. Immunocompromised patients are susceptible to postoperative infections, which may be fatal, in spite of perioperative antibiotic administration. They are also at risk for poor wound healing. Therefore, conservative measures such as bulking agents, sitz baths, and topical analgesics are recommended for patients with severe immunodeficiency. For those patients with mild to moderate immunodeficiency other modalities, such as photocoagulation or injection sclerotherapy, may be considered. This is especially true for patients with leukemia or lymphoma, but not necessarily true for HIV-positive and AIDS patients.

Hewitt et al. [5], in a retrospective study comparing HIV-negative patients with HIV-positive patients (CD4 counts above and below 200 cells/ml) who underwent hemorrhoidectomy, concluded that HIV status should not alter the indications for hemorrhoidectomy. There was no statistical difference in postoperative complications or time to wound healing in either of these groups of patients. In contrast, Morandi et al. [6], in a prospective study comparing wound healing times in HIV-negative, HIV–positive, and AIDS patients undergoing hemorrhoidectomy, found that HIV positivity and the presence of AIDS significantly delayed wound healing and also correlated with the presence of infection. In their study only 66% of HIV-positive patients and none of the AIDS patients had closed wounds after 14 weeks, and after 32 weeks this increased to 100% and 50%, respectively. They concluded that hemorrhoidectomy should be approached with caution in the patient with AIDS, and the CD4 counts and Karnofsky score should be assessed prior to surgery.

Other authors have explored less invasive measures to treat symptomatic hemorrhoids in the HIV+/AIDS population. Scaglia et al. [7] reported on 22 patients with AIDS treated with injection sclerotherapy for symptomatic second-, third-, and fourth-degree hemorrhoids. Some patients required more than one treatment, but treatment was considered to be uncomplicated and successful in all patients. Moore and Fleshner [8], in a retrospective review, demonstrated the safety and efficacy of rubber band ligation for symptomatic hemorrhoids in asymptomatic HIV-positive patients suffering from hemorrhoidal disease.

End-Stage Renal Disease

Patients with end-stage renal disease (ESRD) have characteristic problems of chronic constipation, anemia, uremia, and multiple medical comorbidities. In our practice, Sheikh and colleagues [9] reported on 18 patients with ESRD on dialysis who underwent anorectal surgery. Overall morbidity was 16%, with two patients developing postoperative bleeding and one patient developing intersphincteric abscess. There was no delay in wound healing when compared to patients without renal failure. They recommended dialysis to be performed preoperatively within 24 h of surgery and on postoperative day two with a heparin cover. They concluded that anorectal surgery in the well-managed ESRD patient on dialysis is safe.

Chronic Liver Disease

Chronic liver disease and cirrhosis may result in portal hypertension and subsequent varices of the gastrointestinal tract (including anorectal varices), coagulopathy, and bleeding. It is important to differentiate anorectal varices from bleeding hemorrhoids because the treatment is different. Hemorrhoids are vascular cushions composed of venular and arteriolar anastomoses without communications to the portal venous system. On anoscopic examination, they are purple, usually prolapse into the anoscope, and are not located above the dentate line. In comparison, anorectal varices are collaterals connecting the portal system (superior hemorrhoidal vein) to the systemic circulation (inferior hemorrhoidal vein) [10]. On examination, they are dark blue, extend from the anal verge to the rectum, and do not prolapse into the proctoscope.

Unlike esophageal varices, anorectal varices rarely bleed [11]. Similarly, massive bleeding from prolapsed hemorrhoids in patients with portal hypertension is uncommon. In 1983, Bernstein reviewed the pathophysiology of hemorrhoids and explained that portal hypertension is not the cause of hemorrhoids [12]. Therefore, patients with portal hypertension and active rectal bleeding should be examined with flexible sigmoidoscopy, which is the most reliable method to diagnose anorectal varices [10, 13]. Endoscopic ultrasound with color Doppler has also been recommended in diagnosing anorectal varices. Fantin et al. [10] and Katz et al. [14] describe the use of transjugular intrahepatic portosystemic shunting (TIPS) to control bleeding from anorectal varices.

Massive bleeding from prolapsed hemorrhoids in patients with portal hypertension, although uncommon, may be life-threatening. Anoscopic examination is necessary to identify the site of bleeding. As described by Nivatvongs in [15], the anal canal is anesthetized with 0.25% bupivacaine containing 1:200,000 epinephrine, and a figure-of-eight suture is placed using a 3.0 synthetic absorbable suture. The suture should incorporate the mucosa, submucosa, and internal sphincter in order to achieve hemostasis [15]. Any coagulopathy should be corrected as well. Resuturing of the site may be necessary if rebleeding occurs. Hemorrhoidectomy is reserved only for those cases where suture ligation has failed.

Pregnancy

Hemorrhoids are common during pregnancy. Ledward [16] reported hemorrhoids requiring treatment in 9.3% of women at the time of delivery. Hemorrhoids may be common in pregnant women secondary to several physiologic factors. Constipation is common secondary to high levels of circulating progesterone, mechanical obstruction by the gravid uterus, and as a result of iron supplementation which is a part of prenatal care. Also, circulating blood volume is increased by 25–40% during pregnancy, which may contribute to venous dilation and engorgement.

Treatment of hemorrhoids in pregnancy is based on symptoms, severity of disease, and trimester. External hemorrhoids require treatment for painful or acute thrombosis with local excision only. First- and second-degree internal hemorrhoids may be managed with dietary modification [17]. This should include a high-fiber diet, psyllium seed preparation, and increased fluid intake. If symptoms persist, a minor office procedure such as injection sclerotherapy with 5% phenol in almond oil may be used [17, 18]. There have been no clinical studies reporting on the use of infrared photocoagulation or rubber band ligation in the pregnant patient. However, these have been shown to be effective outpatient procedures for symptomatic hemorrhoids in the nonpregnant patient. One should keep in mind, however, the small risk of perineal sepsis associated with rubber band ligation.

Hemorrhoids complicated by acute thrombosis, strangulation/incarceration of prolapsed internal hemorrhoids, or intractable pain require surgical hemorrhoidectomy. Saleeby et al. [19], from our practice, reported on 25 women, 22 of whom were in the third trimester, who underwent closed hemorrhoidectomy for acute hemorrhoidal crisis. All surgeries were performed in the left Sims' position for women in the third trimester and in the prone jackknife position for all other patients. All surgeries were performed under local anesthesia with intravenous sedation. All patients experienced relief of pain within 24 h, except one patient who required placement of a hemostatic pack in the anal canal for postoperative bleeding. There were no surgery-related fetal complications, and all wounds healed within six weeks.

Surgical hemorrhoidectomy has also been reported to be safe and effective in the immediate postpartum period. Ruiz-Moreno [20] reported no complications after operating on 90 postpartum women on days 0–4 after delivery. Schottler [21] reported on a similar group of women and had a minor complication rate of 3.1% . Both studies show the safety of performing surgical hemorrhoidectomy in the immediate postpartum setting. Women should be advised that hemorrhoids may recur with subsequent pregnancies. Therefore it is usually recommended to postpone hemorrhoidectomy until after a women has completed her childbearing unless there is acute strangulation or thrombus.

The Anticoagulated Patient

This topic is discussed in detail in Chapter 28.

Associated Perianal Disease

When hemorrhoids are associated with other perianal disease processes such as pruritus ani, abscess, etc., the primary disease process should be treated first prior to any surgical hemorrhoidectomy. For example, the abscess should be drained and sufficiently treated.

Hematologic Disorders

Those hematologic disorders in the immunocompromised patient were discussed in the section entitled "Immunosuppression." Another group of patients with hematologic disorders are those with bleeding disorders such as clotting deficiencies (i.e., von Willebrand's disease, thrombocytopenia, etc.). Prager, Khubchandani et al. in 1971 reviewed a series of these patients and reported that anorectal conditions could be treated safely as long as the patients were followed closely, their deficiencies replaced with the help of a hematologist prior to surgery, and the most conservative approach applied (i.e., one quadrant hemorrhoidectomy) in selected patients [22]. In 1989, Orangio and Lucas reported on a patient with hemophilia who developed Factor VIII inhibitors and continued to hemorrhage after routine hemorrhoidectomy [23]. The patient was salvaged with persistent, aggressive, combined medical and surgical therapies which included rectal packing, angiography with embolization, abdominal perineal resection, and massive Factor VIII and Factor IX concentrates, platelet, and fresh frozen plasma transfusions.

References

1. Jeffery PJ, Parks AG, Ritchie JK. Treatment of haemorrhoids in patients with inflammatory bowel disease. Lancet 1977;1:1084–1085.
2. Rankin GB, Watts HD, Clifford S, Melnyk CS, Kellrey ML Jr. National cooperative Crohn's disease study: extraintestinal manifestations and perianal complications. Gastroenterology 1979;77(4):914–920.
3. Homan WP, Tang CK, Thorbjarnarson B. Anal lesions complicating Crohn's disease. Arch Surg 1976;111:1333–1335.
4. Wolkomir AF, Luchtefeld MA. Surgery for symptomatic hemorrhoids and anal fissures in Crohn's disease. Dis Colon Rectum 1993;36(6):545–547.
5. Hewitt RW, Sokol TP, Fleshner PR. Should HIV status alter indications for hemorrhoidectomy? Dis Colon Rectum 1996;39(6):615–618.
6. Morandi E, Merlini D, Salvaggio A, Foschi D, Trabucchi E. Prospective study of healing time after hemorrhoidectomy: influence of HIV infection, acquired immunodeficiency syndrome, and anal wound infection. Dis Colon Rectum 1999;42(9):1140–1144.
7. Scaglia M, Delaini G, Destefano I, Hulten L. Injection treatment of hemorrhoids in patients with acquired immunodeficiency syndrome. Dis Colon Rectum 2001;44(3):401–404.
8. Moore BA, Fleshner PR. Rubber band ligation for hemorrhoidal disease can be safely performed in select HIV-positive patients. Dis Colon Rectum 2001;44(8):1079–1082.
9. Sheikh F, Khubchandani IT, Rosen L, Sheets JA, Stasik JJ. Is anorectal surgery on chronic dialysis patients risky? Dis Colon Rectum 1992;35:56–58.
10. Fantin AC, Risti B, Debatin JF, Schopke W, Meyenberger C. Bleeding anorectal varices: successful treatment with transjugular intrahepatic portosystemic shunting (TIPS). Gut 1996;38:932–935.
11. Nivatvong S. Hemorrhoids. In: Gordon PH, Nivatvongs S. Principles and practice of surgery for the colon, rectum and anus, 3rd ed. Quality Medical Publishing, Inc., 2007:144–166.
12. Bernstein WC. What are hemorrhoids and what is their relationship to the portal venous system? Dis Colon Rectum 1983;26(12):829–834.
13. Herman BE, Baum S, Denobile J, Volpe RJ. Massive bleeding from rectal varices. Am J Gastroenterol 1993;88:939–942.
14. Katz JA, Rubin RA, Cope C, Holland G, Brass CA. Recurrent bleeding from anorectal varices: successful treatment

with a transjugular intrahepatic porto-systemic shunt. Gastroenterology 1993;88:1104–1107.

15. Nivatvongs S. Suture of massive hemorrhoidal bleeding in portal hypertension. Dis Colon Rectum 1985;28: 878–879.

16. Ledward RS. The management of puerperal hemorrhoids: a double-blind clinical trial of Anacal rectal ointment. Practitioner 1980;224:660–661.

17. Medich DS, Fazio VW. Hemorrhoids, anal fissure, and carcinoma of the colon, rectum, and anus during pregnancy. Surg Clin N Am 1995;75(1):77–88.

18. Simmons SL. Anorectal disorders in pregnancy. J Obstet Gynecol 1964;71:960–962.

19. Saleeby RG, Rosen L, Stasik JJ, Riether RD, Sheets J, Khubchandani IT. Hemorrhoidectomy during pregnancy: risk or relief? Dis Colon Rectum 1991;34:260–261.

20. Ruiz-Moreno F. Surgery in the puerperium for painful anorectal disorders. Proc Soc Med 1970;63:102–103.

21. Schottler JL, Balcus EC, Goldberg SM. Postpartum hemorrhoidectomy. Dis Colon Rectum 1973;16:395–396.

22. Prager D, Khubchandani IT, Trimpi HD, Martin PV. Proctologic disorders and hematologic diseases. Dis Colon Rectum 1971;14(1):4–11.

23. Orangio GR, Lucas GW. Management of hemophilia in colon and rectal surgery. Dis Colon Rectum 1989;32(10): 878–883.

23 Ambulatory Hemorrhoidectomy

Daniel O. Herzig and H. Randolph Bailey

Symptomatic hemorrhoids are one of the oldest described afflictions of humans. Treatment has evolved over time, but hemorrhoidectomy remains an option recommended to many patients. Among the advances in the treatment of hemorrhoids in recent years, one of the most significant has been the shift from the inpatient to the outpatient setting. This chapter outlines the principles of hemorrhoidectomy in the ambulatory setting.

Evolution of Ambulatory Hemorrhoidectomy

Ambulatory (day-stay) hemorrhoidectomy provides substantial cost benefit to the health care system. The UK Department of Health's National Health Service Plan (2000) set a target that 75% of elective procedures should be day cases. Hemorrhoidectomy is one of 25 procedures cited in the plan as suitable for day-stay. Despite this recommendation, the number of day-stay cases in the UK has not risen as quickly as anticipated. A recent report by the Healthcare Commission examined the reasons for this slow rise in day surgical procedures [1]. Data from the Healthcare Commission, reported from Hospital Episode Statistics (HES), showed the baseline rate of day-stay hemorrhoidectomy in 1998–1999 was slightly less than 10%. It was considered to be

"rising from a low base." In addition to a sizeable worldwide experience with ambulatory hemorrhoidectomy, day-stay hemorrhoidectomy has also been studied within the UK healthcare system [2]. The introduction of specific guidelines for patient selection and appropriate use of day-stay hemorrhoidectomy in the UK have been shown to substantially improve its rate of utilization [3]. Nevertheless, in the most current NHS data, the rate of day-stay hemorrhoidectomy was still only 30% for 2005–2006. While substantially improved, this proportion is still quite low relative to American standards.

A recent informal survey at the American Society of Colon and Rectal Surgeons annual meeting cited over 75% of hemorrhoidectomy procedures being done in an outpatient setting. The concept of ambulatory hemorrhoidectomy has been widely embraced in the US for some time. More than 20 years ago, Smith proposed that over 90% of anorectal procedures could be performed on an outpatient basis [4]. According to the National Center for Health Statistics, ambulatory surgical procedures accounted for 63% of all American community hospital operations in 2002, compared with 16% in 1980 [5]. However, nearly one-half of these are ophthalmologic or gastrointestinal endoscopic procedures. In response to the growing acceptance of ambulatory anorectal surgery, the American Society of Colon and Rectal Surgeons published practice parameters in 2003, outlining accepted principles for outpatient care [6]. Ambulatory

I. Khubchandani et al. (eds.), *Surgical Treatment of Hemorrhoids*, DOI 10.1007/978-1-84800-314-9_23,
© Springer-Verlag London Limited 2009

hemorrhoidectomy continues to be performed with increasing frequency worldwide as its role becomes better defined [7, 8, 9, 10, 11, 12, 13, 14, 15, 16, 17, 18, 19].

Preoperative Considerations

The paramount preoperative consideration is patient selection. Most hemorrhoidal disease does not require any treatment in the operating room. Bleday and associates reported their experience in Minneapolis with over 22,000 patient visits for complicated hemorrhoids [20]. They found that nonoperative management was suitable treatment for nearly 90% of this large cohort. Of those patients treated without an operation, half responded to conservative measures and half were successfully managed with office rubber band ligation. This has been our experience as well, because we treat only a small minority of patients with symptomatic hemorrhoids with excisional hemorrhoidectomy. Appropriate patients for hemorrhoidectomy include those with disease refractory to office procedures, patients unable to tolerate office procedures, patients with significant external hemorrhoids, patients with Grade III internal hemorrhoids after failure of rubber band ligation, and those with Grade IV internal/external hemorrhoids refractory to dietary measures and office treatments [21, 22].

Once the decision to proceed with hemorrhoidectomy has been made, appropriate evaluation of the patient's medical condition is necessary. Prerequisites to ambulatory surgery include appropriate transportation to and from the hospital, the presence of a responsible adult to assist in the patient's care for the first 24 h postoperatively, and the ability for the patient to contact the surgical team should problems arise. Preoperative education of the patient is critical to the success of ambulatory hemorrhoidectomy. Discussion includes a reasonable expectation for pain as well as management of multiple issues of importance. Detailed written instructions are provided which deal with pain control,

prevention and management of urinary retention, and regulation of bowel movements.

A thorough history and physical exam is necessary for all patients. The American Society of Anesthesiology (ASA) classification system offers a simple scale as an initial consideration [23]. The ASA classification system is a validated predictor of morbidity and mortality after operation [24, 25]. Patients who meet criteria for ASA class I or II are generally considered safe to proceed with ambulatory surgery. Some patients who fall into ASA class III but have well-compensated and stable disease may still be selectively offered outpatient therapy.

Cardiac risk evaluation can be performed in accordance with American College of Cardiology/American Heart Association guidelines [26]. These guidelines stratify patients on the basis of their baseline risk coupled with their functional capacity and the type of procedure they are to undergo. Hemorrhoidectomy is considered a low risk procedure. Therefore, the chance of cardiac complications is low unless the patient has major clinical predictors such as myocardial infarction within 6 months, decompensated congestive heart failure, a significant arrhythmia, or severe valvular disease. If any of these elements are present, additional cardiac testing is warranted. No other routine tests are ordered except that all women of childbearing age should have a pregnancy test. Additional noncardiac testing should be directed at evaluation of specific symptoms or signs of underlying illness [27].

Mechanical or antibiotic bowel preparation is generally not needed prior to hemorrhoidectomy. However, to reduce the risk of postoperative fecal impaction, it is reasonable for the patient to administer a phosphate or saline enema prior to the procedure.

Preoperative antibiotics are unproven for prophylaxis of anorectal infection. While guidelines for prophylaxis for colon resection are well-described, similar recommendations do not exist for anorectal procedures [28]. Consideration could be given to prophylaxis in the elderly, severe diabetics, or patients with immune dysfunction. For these patients, antibiotics similar to those used for prophylaxis prior to colon resection can be used, such as second generation cephalosporin, cephazolin, and metronidazole, or ertapenem. For those with a penicillin allergy, a fluoroquinolone and metronidazole may be used [28]. Recent revisions to the guidelines for endocarditis prophylaxis have been published by the American Heart Association. Administration of antibiotics solely to prevent endocarditis is not recommended for patients who undergo a genitourinary or gastrointestinal tract procedure[29]. Because of the short duration of the operation and early postoperative ambulation, there is generally no need for DVT prophylaxis with hemorrhoidectomy.

Intra-Operative Considerations

No single advance has had a greater effect in facilitating ambulatory hemorrhoidectomy than the effective provision of anesthesia. Pain following hemorrhoidectomy has been perhaps the greatest obstacle preventing more widespread use of ambulatory hemorrhoidectomy. However, improvements in general, regional, and local anesthesia, as well as postoperative oral analgesics, have resulted in adequate pain control for the majority of patients.

Multiple anesthesia techniques have been described for ambulatory hemorrhoidectomy. General endotracheal, general by laryngeal mask airway, epidural, spinal, and local with sedation are all options. Coordination of care with an anesthesiologist is essential to minimize perioperative morbidity. This starts with agreement on positioning, either prone jackknife or lithotomy. Some surgeons are quite emotional in their support for a particular position for anorectal operations. While surgeons may prefer sedation and local anesthesia, many anesthesiologists are uncomfortable managing deep sedation with a patient in the prone position. A compromise is often required. Read and colleagues reviewed their experience with deep sedation and prone positioning [30]. Of 389 patients who underwent anorectal procedures in the prone position, 260 (67%) received intravenous sedation plus local anesthesia, 125 (32%) received regional anesthesia (spinal or epidural), and 4 (1%) received general endotracheal anesthesia. Forty-two adverse events attributable to the anesthetic occurred in 18 patients: nausea and vomiting (n = 17), transient hypotension, bradycardia, or arrhythmia (n = 8), transient hypoxia or hypoventilation (n = 7), urinary retention (n = 6), and severe patient discomfort (n = 2). The complication rate was the same in the local/sedation group and the regional anesthesia group. Recovery time before discharge for patients treated on an ambulatory basis was significantly shorter for those patients undergoing intravenous sedation plus local anesthesia. We generally avoid regional anesthesia because of the small risk of spinal headache, the additional time required for its administration, and the frequent need for additional IV fluid administration due to the vasodilation in the lower extremities.

It is our preference to perform these procedures with the patient in lithotomy position. Lithotomy position gives excellent exposure for the majority of patients [31, 32, 33]. Furthermore, sedation is easily managed, and the anesthesia team has continuous and ready access to the airway, avoiding the need for endotracheal intubation in most patients. Adequate relaxation is provided with deep sedation or general anesthesia by way of a laryngeal mask airway. Induction times are shorter, there is little time and energy spent rolling the patient, and there is less chance for positioning injuries. Nerve injuries, principally obturator, or lateral femoral cutaneous nerve injuries, are rarely reported and are virtually never seen with operation times less than 2 h [34]. Using candy cane stirrups allows for hip flexion during positioning, negating any strain on the obturator nerves [35].

Once the patient is in position—and regardless of whether sedation, regional, or general anesthesia is used—it is important to provide a perianal block for sphincter relaxation and postoperative analgesia. Even for a patient under general anesthesia, the benefits of an anal block will be readily apparent upon emergence from anesthesia. Local perianal block is well established and effective [32, 36, 37, 38, 39, 40] Argov reported his personal experience of 2,245 ambulatory hemorrhoidectomies over two decades [10]. He describes using a local anal block so effectively as to require only low dose midazolam as the single additional medication.

Additional postoperative analgesia can be obtained by the use of an intravenous nonsteroidal anti-inflammatory medication (NSAID) (in patients without a bleeding diathesis, peptic ulcer disease, or renal dysfunction) [41]. This agent can be given intravenously, intramuscularly, or even directly into the sphincter muscle. The simplest route of administration is IV at the end of the procedure. The principal advantage of the NSAID is to provide an analgesic effect and to reduce the need for opioids. In the US, ketorolac is the only available intravenous NSAID; it is approved for oral use as well. Significant reductions in urinary retention have been reported with the use of ketorolac [42]. It is continued in our patients for 5 days postoperatively as a scheduled medication. (See additional details about postoperative analgesia below.)

Particular attention should be paid to the amount of intravenous fluid administered, to prevent urinary retention. Once the intravenous catheter is placed, care should be taken to minimize preoperative infusion, which is best done by not attaching an infusion bag to the intravenous catheter. In the operating room, the anesthesia staff should give only the amount of fluid required to safely administer medications. There are few, if any, reasons for the total amount of fluid infused to exceed 100–200 ml for the perioperative period. The role of excessive fluid administration in postoperative urinary retention is well-reported, but these data may not be familiar to many anesthesiologists.

Technical Considerations

The technique for hemorrhoidectomy has been extensively described by others [43, 44]. We prefer the closed, Ferguson-type, hemorrhoidectomy. Our preference for this technique is to use deep sedation or a light general anesthetic, with the patient in lithotomy position. A long-acting local anesthetic (e.g., bupivicaine) with epinephrine is used. If the patient is lightly sedated, adding

bicarbonate may reduce the discomfort of injection. A dermal perianal field block is provided by injecting anesthetic in a diamond shape beyond the external hemorrhoidal tissue for the superficial injection. Additional anesthetic is then infiltrated in the area of the pudendal nerve, medial and posterior to the ischial tuberosities. Finally, the remaining anesthetic is injected through a needle guided in the intersphincteric groove towards the submucosa of the rectal ampulla, with additional anesthetic provided on withdrawal. This provides substantial and long-acting analgesia with excellent muscle relaxation of the sphincter to aid in exposure. The epinephrine also reduces oozing during the procedure and makes the operative planes easier to define.

Multiple energy sources have been described for assistance with dissection [45, 46, 47, 48, 49, 50, 51]. While some statistically significant differences have been reported, we do not feel the level of clinical benefit warrants the higher costs. After an anal block is performed, a four-quadrant anoscopic exam is carried out, and an operative plan is made regarding how many hemorrhoids require excision. The specific details of the Ferguson hemorrhoidectomy are omitted here but can be found elsewhere in this textbook.

The introduction of a circular mucosal resection and stapled hemorrhoidopexy (procedure for prolapse and hemorrhoids, PPH) was first described by Longo in 1998 [52]. Since then, considerable data have been acquired regarding the effectiveness of this procedure [53, 54]. Most of the studies have shown less postoperative pain with the PPH procedure, possibly making it attractive as an ambulatory procedure [55–57].

While multiple and extensive benefits of PPH have been reported, so have profound complications [58, 59, 60, 61]. Because of these cautionary notes, and after caring for patients with similar complications, we have come to perform this procedure infrequently. We find PPH to be most effective for circumferential internal hemorrhoids, but many of these patients also tend to respond well to sequential rubber band ligation. For those with more extensive internal and external disease, it is preferable in our opinion to proceed with excisional hemorrhoidectomy to treat both the internal and external components.

Postoperative Considerations

Patients recover for about 30–60 min before discharge from the facility. Some surgeons consider discharging the patient in 23 h to be an ambulatory procedure. We strongly favor early discharge while the local anesthetic is still in effect. A "post-anesthesia discharge score" (PADS) is recorded when considering discharge (see Table 23.1). They are allowed to leave if the PADS score is at least 9. Specifically, patients are not required to urinate prior to discharge. They are told that with fluid restriction, their bladders may not fill for 12–18 h after the operation. They must have a responsible adult take them home. It is recommended that they have assistance at home for at least the first night after the operation. Patients are given written discharge instructions which include guidance about pain control, bowel movements, dealing with difficulty voiding, and minor bleeding, and when to call. A 24-h telephone number is given to contact the surgical team with any questions or problems.

Table 23.1 Post-Anesthesia Discharge Scoring System

Vital Signs
  2 = Within 20% of preoperative value
  1 = 20–40% of preoperative value
  0 = 40% of preoperative value
Ambulatory and Mental Status
  2 = Oriented times 3 and has a steady gait
  1 = Oriented times 3 or has steady gait
  0 = Neither
Pain or Nausea/Vomiting
  2 = Minimal
  1 = Moderate
  0 = Severe
Surgical Bleeding
  2 = Minimal
  1 = Moderate
  0 = Severe
Intake and Output
  2 = Has had PO fluids and voided
  1 = Has had PO fluids or voided
  0 = Neither
Total score is 10. Patients scoring 9 or more are considered fit for discharge.

Pain and urinary retention are the most common issues complicating recovery from ambulatory hemorrhoidectomy [62]. The incidence of urinary retention has been reported at 1–50% [62, 63, 64, 65, 66, 67]. The Mayo Clinic reported their rate at 34% following hemorrhoidectomy, with independent risk factors being three- or four-quadrant excisions, morphine equivalents >33 mg, and male gender [63]. The amount of fluid given during hemorrhoidectomy is also directly correlated with urinary retention [64, 66, 67, 68]. Bailey and Ferguson reported a reduction in urinary retention from 15% to 4% using a combination of a restrictive fluid strategy and delaying bladder catheterization until the bladder is full [67]. The underlying cause of urinary retention is not known, but may be due to pelvic muscle spasm, detrusor dysfunction, bladder outlet dysfunction, or pain [64, 65, 69]. There is some evidence to suggest that ambulatory hemorrhoidectomy results in a lower rate of urinary retention, since the total amount of fluids administered is reduced [66]. Ambulatory patients also do not have the additional psychological stress produced by the nurse's inquiring every hour if they have voided! As noted earlier, significant reductions in urinary retention have been reported with the use of ketorolac [42].

We have found a combination of methods to substantially lower the rate of urinary retention. Patients have nothing to eat or drink after midnight before the operation. Once at the ambulatory surgical suite, an intravenous catheter is placed and capped. When the patient is taken to the operating room, a small (250 ml) bag of crystalloid is attached using "minidrip" tubing (tubing which allows 60 drops/ml, as opposed to the standard 10 drops/ml). After induction, the total amount of fluid is kept to a safe minimum except for medications, and then stopped after the procedure. The patient is not even asked to urinate prior to discharge. The patient is instructed to maintain minimal liquid intake (<250 ml) until urinating. If after several hours the patient is unable to void spontaneously, we recommend that they try a warm tub bath to relax the pelvic floor and allow voiding. The patient is encouraged, if necessary, to try to urinate while in the tub. The warm bath may allow enough pelvic floor relaxation to allow micturition.

Pain is one of the most feared complications after ambulatory hemorrhoidectomy. It is important for patients to expect some discomfort and to schedule an adequate recovery period away from their work. Patient education and reassurance often go a long way in alleviating anxiety and pain. Patients undergoing PPH can expect lower pain scores (by about 40%) and a 35–40% reduction in the amount of analgesics needed [53]. Pain on the day of the procedure is usually minimal due to the long-acting perianal block and the administration of an intravenous NSAID as described above. We prescribe an additional five days of scheduled ketorolac (10 mg q 6 h). In addition, an oral opioid is prescribed on an as-needed basis. The most commonly prescribed form of oral opioid is a combination of hydrocodone and acetaminophen. The limiting ingredient in this combination is the acetaminophen, usually 500 mg per 5 mg of hydrocodone. Other preparations with less acetaminophen (325/5 mg hydrocodone) allow the patient to take more of the opioid. Substantial pain relief can often be achieved with a warm tub bath (sitz bath). This can be done as often as the patient likes without harm to wound healing. We recommend tub soaks for 10–15 min three or more times per day to relax muscle spasm, promote drainage, and assist healing. Most pain is markedly better after the first week. The majority of patients are off analgesics within two weeks of the procedure. In the absence of a specific issue, the first planned postoperative visit to the office is 2–3 weeks after the procedure.

Fecal impaction can be a serious problem after hemorrhoidectomy and may require operative intervention for disimpaction. Clearly, the best treatment for this is prevention. Patients are instructed to begin a fiber supplement (psyllium) with water the morning after the operation. Once they are voiding satisfactorily, patients are encouraged to drink ample fluids (at least 64 ounces of water or juice each day). Written instructions are provided to avoid constipation: If there is no bowel movement by the evening of the first postoperative day, 30 ml of milk of magnesia is taken. If there is no bowel movement by

the next morning, milk of magnesia is then repeated. If there is no bowel movement by the morning of the third postoperative day, half a bottle (about 150 ml) of magnesium citrate is taken and is repeated in the afternoon if no result. By the morning of the fourth postoperative day, if none of the above has worked, the patient is instructed to contact the office. While some patients have disregarded these directions and become impacted, we rarely see impactions in those who have followed this plan. Most patients should stay on fiber after the operation for as long as they can be compliant. While taking the opioid analgesics, we suggest an evening dose of milk of magnesia each day the patient does not have a bowel movement.

Minor bleeding is generally self-limited. More substantial bleeding, either immediately after the operation or delayed, may require reoperation. Patients should be seen and evaluated in the event of significant bleeding. Patients should avoid heavy lifting and straining. We advise that patients avoid driving for as long as they require opioid analgesics. There are very few other restrictions which are practical or necessary. Patients will generally restrict themselves more than the surgeon recommends.

Conclusions

Ambulatory hemorrhoidectomy is a safe and effective procedure when indicated. It is appropriate for the majority of patients requiring hemorrhoidectomy. Pain, urinary retention and other complications can be minimized and, for the most part, be managed outside the hospital. Medical comorbidities are the most substantial obstacle for outpatient surgery. Patients with severe medical illnesses may require a hospital stay for issues unrelated to the operation. For those patients who are suitable for ambulatory hemorrhoidectomy, it is imperative that there is appropriate assistance from caregivers at home and that there is a clear and reliable method for the patient to contact the surgical team with any questions or problems.

References

1. Commission for Healthcare Audit and Inspection. Acute hospital portfolio review: day surgery. Commission for Healthcare Audit and Inspection, 2005.
2. Hunt L, Luck AJ, Rudkin G, Hewett PJ. Day-case haemorrhoidectomy. Br J Surg 1999;86:255–8.
3. Heer R, Dobson D, Plusa SM. How to alter surgical practice? The use of guidelines to encourage day-case haemorrhoidectomy. J R Coll Surg Edinb 2000;45:369–70.
4. Smith LE. Ambulatory surgery for anorectal diseases: an update. South Med J 1986;79:163–166.
5. National Center for Health Statistics. Health, United States, 2004.
6. Place R, Hyman N, Simmang C et al. Practice parameters for ambulatory anorectal surgery. Dis Colon Rectum 2003; 46:573–6.
7. Tjandra JJ. Ambulatory haemorrhoidectomy—has the time come? ANZ J Surg 2005;75:183.
8. Altomare DF, Roveran A, Pecorella G, Gaj F, Stortini E. The treatment of hemorrhoids: guidelines of the Italian Society of Colorectal Surgery. Tech Coloproctol 2006; 10:181–6.
9. Argov S. Ambulatory radical hemorrhoidectomy: personal experience with 1,530 Milligan-Morgan operations with follow-up of 2–15 years. Dig Surg 1999;16:375–8.
10. Argov S, Levandovsky O. Radical, ambulatory hemorrhoidectomy under local anesthesia. Am J Surg 2001; 182:69–72.
11. Carditello A. Ambulatory hemorrhoidectomy: results of 500 surgical operations. Chir Ital 1994;46:68–70.
12. Carditello A, Stilo F. Haemorrhoidectomy according to Ferguson in day-surgery. Experience and results. Ann Ital Chir 2006;77:47–50.
13. Gawenda M, Walter M. Surgical therapy of advanced hemorrhoidal disease—is an ambulatory surgery intervention possible? Chirurg 1996;67:940–3.
14. Ho YH, Lee J, Salleh I, Leong A, Eu KW, Seow-Choen F. Randomized controlled trial comparing same-day discharge with hospital stay following haemorrhoidectomy. Aust N Z J Surg 1998;68:334–6.
15. Kecherukov AI, Ziganhin RV, Aliev FS. Outpatient surgical treatment of hemorrhoids. Khirurgiia (Mosk) 1994;11: 26–9.
16. Labas P, Ohradka B, Cambal M, Olejnik J, Fillo J. Haemorrhoidectomy in outpatient practice. Eur J Surg 2002;168:619–20.
17. Lam TY, Lam SC, Kwok SP. Feasibility case-controlled study of day-case haemorrhoidectomy. [See comment]. ANZ J Surg 2001;71:652–4.
18. Robinson AM, Smith LE, Perciballi JA. Outpatient hemorrhoidectomy. Mil Med 1990;155:299–300.
19. Takano M. Day surgery for anal disease. Nippon Geka Gakkai Zasshi 2000;101:733–40.
20. Bleday R, Pena JP, Rothenberger DA, Goldberg SM, Buls JG. Symptomatic hemorrhoids: current incidence and complications of operative therapy. Dis Colon Rectum 1992;35:477–481.
21. Cataldo P, Ellis CN, Gregorcyk S et al. Practice parameters for the management of hemorrhoids (revised). Dis Colon Rectum 2005;48:189–94.
22. MacRae HM, McLeod RS. Comparison of hemorrhoidal treatment modalities. A meta-analysis. Dis Colon Rectum 1995;38:687–94.
23. ASA. New classification of physical status. Anesthesiology 1963;24:111.
24. Menke H, Klein A, John KD, Junginger T. Predictive value of ASA classification for the assessment of the perioperative risk. Int Surg 1993;78:266–70.
25. Vacanti CJ, VanHouten RJ, Hill RC. A statistical analysis of the relationship of physical status to postoperative mortality in 68,388 cases. Anesth Analg 1970;49:564–6.
26. Eagle KA, Berger PB, Calkins H et al. ACC/AHA guideline update for perioperative cardiovascular evaluation for noncardiac surgery—executive summary: a report of the American College of Cardiology/American Heart Association Task Force on Practice Guidelines (Committee to Update the 1996 Guidelines on Perioperative Cardiovascular Evaluation for Noncardiac Surgery). J Am Coll Cardiol 2002;39:542–53.
27. Allison JG, Bromley HR. Unnecessary preoperative investigations: evaluation and cost analysis. Am Surg 1996; 62:686–9.
28. Bratzler DW, Houck PM, Surgical Infection Prevention Guidelines Writers Workgroup et al. Antimicrobial prophylaxis for surgery: an advisory statement from the National Surgical Infection Prevention Project. Clin Infect Dis 2004;38:1706–15.
29. Wilson W, Taubert KA, Gewitz M et al. Prevention of infective endocarditis. Guidelines From the American Heart Association. A Guideline from the American Heart Association Rheumatic Fever, Endocarditis, and Kawasaki Disease Committee, Council on Cardiovascular Disease in the Young, and the Council on Clinical Cardiology, Council on Cardiovascular Surgery and Anesthesia, and the Quality of Care and Outcomes Research Interdisciplinary Working Group. Circulation. 2007 Apr 19;[published electronically ahead of print].
30. Read TE, Henry SE, Hovis RM et al. Prospective evaluation of anesthetic technique for anorectal surgery. Dis Colon Rectum 2002;45:1553–8.
31. Bailey HR. The Dorsal lithotomy position: preferred by surgeon and anesthesiologist. In: Bailey HR, Snyder MJ (eds). Ambulatory colon and rectal surgery. New York: Springer Verlag, 1999:51–5.
32. Nivatvongs S. An improved technique of local anesthesia for anorectal surgery. Dis Colon Rectum 1982;25:259–60.
33. Nivatvongs S, Fang DT, Kennedy HL. The shape of the buttocks. A useful guide for selection of anesthesia and patient position in anorectal surgery. Dis Colon Rectum 1983;26:85–6.
34. Warner MA, Warner DO, Harper CM, Schroeder DR, Maxson PM. Lower extremity neuropathies associated with lithotomy positions. Anesthesiology 2000;93:938–42.
35. Litwiller JP, Wells RE Jr, Halliwill JR, Carmichael SW, Warner MA. Effect of lithotomy positions on strain of the obturator and lateral femoral cutaneous nerves. Clin Anat 2004;17:45–9.
36. Gerjy R, Derwinger K, Nystrom PO. Perianal local block for stapled anopexy. Dis Colon Rectum 2006;49:1914–21.
37. Nystrom PO, Derwinger K, Gerjy R. Local perianal block for anal surgery. Tech Coloproctol 2004;8:23–6.
38. Delikoukos S, Zacharoulis D, Hatzitheofilou C. Local posterior perianal block for proctologic surgery. Int Surg 2006;91:348–51.

39. Sobrado CW, Habr-Gama A. Hook-needle puncture. A new technique of local anesthesia for anorectal surgery. Dis Colon Rectum 1996;39:1330–1.

40. Roxas MF, Delima MG. Randomized controlled trial to determine the effectiveness of the Nivatvongs technique versus conventional local anaesthetic infiltration for outpatient haemorrhoidectomy. Asian J Surg 2006;29:70–3.

41. Richman IM. Use of Toradol in anorectal surgery. Dis Colon Rectum 1993;36:295–6.

42. O'Donovan S, Ferrara A, Larach S, Williamson P. Intraoperative use of Toradol facilitates outpatient hemorrhoidectomy. Dis Colon Rectum 1994;37:793–9.

43. Milligan ETC, Morgan CN, Jones LE. Surgical anatomy of the anal canal and operative treatment of haemorrhoids. Lancet 1937;1:1119–1124.

44. Ferguson JA, Heaton JR. Closed hemorrhoidectomy. Dis Colon Rectum 1959;2:176.

45. Jayne DG, Botterill I, Ambrose NS, Brennan TG, Guillou PJ, O'Riordain DS. Randomized clinical trial of Ligasure versus conventional diathermy for day-case haemorrhoidectomy. Br J Surg 2002;89:428–32.

46. Kwok SY, Chung CC, Tsui KK, Li MK. A double-blind, randomized trial comparing Ligasure and Harmonic Scalpel hemorrhoidectomy. Dis Colon Rectum 2005;48:344–8.

47. Chung CC, Ha JP, Tai YP, Tsang WW, Li MK. Double-blind, randomized trial comparing Harmonic Scalpel hemorrhoidectomy, bipolar scissors hemorrhoidectomy, and scissors excision: ligation technique. Dis Colon Rectum 2002;45:789–94.

48. Franklin EJ, Seetharam S, Lowney J, Horgan PG. Randomized, clinical trial of Ligasure vs. conventional diathermy in hemorrhoidectomy. Dis Colon Rectum 2003;46:1380–3.

49. Thorbeck CV, Montes MF. Haemorrhoidectomy: randomised controlled clinical trial of Ligasure compared with Milligan-Morgan operation. Eur J Surg 2002;168:482–4.

50. Armstrong DN, Ambroze WL, Schertzer ME, Orangio GR. Harmonic Scalpel vs. electrocautery hemorrhoidectomy: a prospective evaluation. Dis Colon Rectum 2001; 44:558–64.

51. Palazzo FF, Francis DL, Clifton MA. Randomized clinical trial of Ligasure versus open haemorrhoidectomy. Br J Surg 2002;89:154–7.

52. Longo A. Treatment of hemorrhoids disease by reduction of mucosa and hemorrhoidal prolapse with a circular suturing device: a new procedure. Proceedings of the 6th world congress of endoscopic surgery, 1998:777–784.

53. Tjandra JJ, Chan MKY. Systematic review on the procedure for prolapse and hemorrhoids (stapled hemorrhoidopexy). Dis Colon Rectum 2007;50:878–892.

54. Senagore AJ, Singer M, Abcarian H et al. A prospective, randomized, controlled multicenter trial comparing stapled hemorrhoidopexy and Ferguson hemorrhoidectomy: perioperative and one-year results. Dis Colon Rectum 2004;47:1824–1836.

55. Kairaluoma M, Nuorva K, Kellokumpu I. Day-case stapled (circular) vs. diathermy hemorrhoidectomy. Dis Colon Rectum 2003;46:93–99.

56. Ravo B, Amato A, Bianco V et al. Complications after stapled hemorrhoidectomy: can they be prevented? Tech Coloproctol 2002;6:83–8.

57. Jayaraman S, Colquhoun PH, Malthaner RA. Stapled versus conventional surgery for hemorrhoids. Cochrane Database Syst Rev 2006;(4):CD005393.

58. Cheetham MJ, Cohen CR, Kamm MA, Phillips RK. A randomized, controlled trial of diathermy hemorrhoidectomy vs. stapled hemorrhoidectomy in an intended day-care setting with longer-term follow-up. Dis Colon Rectum 2003;46:491–497.

59. Pescatori M. Stapled hemorrhoidectomy: a word of caution. Int J Colorectal Dis 2002;17:362–3.

60. Ripetti V, Caricato M, Arullani A. Rectal perforation, retropneumoperitoneum, and pneumomediastinum after stapling procedure for prolapsed hemorrhoids: report of a case and subsequent considerations. Dis Colon Rectum 2002;45:268–70.

61. Molloy RG, Kingsmore D. Life threatening pelvic sepsis after stapled haemorrhoidectomy. Lancet 2000;355:810.

62. Toyonaga T, Matsushima M, Sogawa N et al. Postoperative urinary retention after surgery for benign anorectal disease: potential risk factors and strategy for prevention. Int J Colorectal Dis 2006;21:676–82.

63. Zaheer S, Reilly WT, Pemberton JH, Ilstrup D. Urinary retention after operations for benign anorectal diseases. Dis Colon Rectum 1998;41:696–704.

64. Tammela T. Postoperative urinary retention—why the patient cannot void. Scand J Urol Nephrol Suppl 1995;175:75–7.

65. Pompeius R. Detrusor inhibition induced from anal region in man. Acta Chir Scand Suppl 1966;361:1–54.

66. Hoff SD, Bailey HR, Butts DR et al. Ambulatory surgical hemorrhoidectomy—a solution to postoperative urinary retention? Dis Colon Rectum 1994;37:1242–4.

67. Bailey HR, Ferguson JA. Prevention of urinary retention by fluid restriction following anorectal operations. Dis Colon Rectum 1976;19:250–2.

68. Toyonaga T, Matsushima M, Sogawa N et al. Postoperative urinary retention after surgery for benign anorectal disease: potential risk factors and strategy for prevention. Int J Colorectal Dis 2006;21:676–82.

69. Barone JG, Cummings KB. Etiology of acute urinary retention following benign anorectal surgery. Am Surg 1994;60:210–1.

24 Transanal Hemorrhoidal Dearterialization

Pier Paolo Dal Monte

The LORD will smite thee with the botch of Egypt, and with the Hemorrhoids, and with the scab, and with the itch, whereof thou canst not be healed.

Deuteronomy 28:27

Introduction

The history of hemorrhoidal surgery dates back to the ancient Egyptians [1].

In ancient Greece, Hippocrates' treatises provided detailed descriptions of clinical aspects and surgical procedures for hemorrhoids: "One may cut, resect, suture, or burn hemorrhoids. These measures seem to be terrible but they don't cause any damage" [2].

In the 19th century , hemorrhoidal surgery began to be scientifically codified: Frederick Salmon (the founder of St. Mark's hospital) described the mucocutaneous ligation-excision of hemorrhoidal cushions [3], and Whitehead the circular excision of the whole hemorrhoidal area [4].

Currently the most common excision-ligation procedures are the "open hemorrhoidectomy," described in 1937 by Milligan, Morgan, Jones, and Officer [5], and the closed variant of the latter, the Ferguson operation, described in 1959 [6]. These procedures are usually performed as inpatient treatments, and they are generally burdened by severe postoperative pain. For this reason less invasive outpatient treatments have been developed, such as rubber band ligation [7, 8], infrared coagulation [9], and sclerotherapy [10]. The first one, in particular,

became very popular for its good results and low complication rate in second-degree symptomatic piles [11]. The main disadvantages of these outpatient procedures are the necessity of several treatments and the high recurrence rate (depending upon the hemorrhoidal stage) [12, 13, 14].

The surgical management of hemorrhoids has changed over the last decade. The technique of stapled hemorrhoidopexy, introduced by Longo [15], is a less painful alternative to traditional surgery. In 1995 Morinaga described a new technique for the surgical treatment of hemorrhoids: this technique consists of ligation of the terminal branches of the superior rectal artery in order to eliminate the hemorrhoidal symptoms. He utilized a proctoscope coupled with a Doppler probe to locate and ligate those arteries, reporting good results for this technique [16].

Rationale

The hemorrhoidal cushions consist of plexuses of large venous spaces, arterio-venous communications between the terminal branches of the superior rectal arteries and the superior, middle, and inferior rectal vein [17, 18, 19, 20]. These structures

I. Khubchandani et al. (eds.), *Surgical Treatment of Hemorrhoids*, DOI 10.1007/978-1-84800-314-9_24,
© Springer-Verlag London Limited 2009

have been named by Stelzner as corpus cavernosum recti (CCR) [21]. The blood supply to the CCR is provided by the terminal branches of the superior rectal artery; it is a functional blood supply that fills this cavernous network [22, 23, 24, 25, 26]. This structure plays an important role in continence by acting as a conformable plug, in order to ensure the complete closure of the anal canal. This mechanism contributes up to 15–20% of resting anal pressure [27, 28, 29, 30, 31].

Even though the pathogenesis of hemorrhoids is not completely explained [32, 33, 34, 35], there are two major theories that do not exclude each other: the sliding down theory and the vascular theory. The first assumes that prolapsed hemorrhoids are caused by a pathological slippage of the normal anal lining, caused by the deterioration of supportive connective tissue and increased by the straining during defecation [17, 20, 33,35,]. The second, the "vascular hyperplasia theory," supposes that an abnormal behaviour of the arterio-venous shunt is responsible for the hypertension of hemorrhoidal plexuses, their consequent dilatation, and therefore their prolapse and bleeding [19, 38, 39, 40].

In reality the etiopathogenesis of the hemorrhoidal disease is multifactorial and either of the two theories alone is not sufficient to explain all its aspects. Several studies have demonstrated high resting anal pressure in patients. It is presumed that this high pressure is caused by increased activity of the internal anal sphincter [41, 42, 43, 44] or the external anal sphincter [38, 39], or by increased vascular pressure within the anal cushions [24, 25, 26, 27, 28, 29, 30, 31, 32, 33, 34, 35, 36, 37, 38, 39, 40]. The deterioration with age of the supportive connective tissue causes a lack of support of the blood vessels within the hemorrhoidal plexuses [17, 20, 32, 34, 35] that facilitates the hypertension of the anal cushions [24, 40]. This leads to increased straining during defecation that impairs the venous drainage and facilitates a further increase of cushion pressure with a stress on the connective supportive mesh, finally resulting in intermittent or permanent prolapse [17, 20, 32] (Table 24.1).

The ideal surgical technique for hemorrhoidal disease should consider and have efficacy on both mechanisms, with regard to anatomy and physiology. The excision techniques are very effective because they remove the whole hemorrhoidal plexuses, ligating the vascular pedicles. This approach is far from being physiological, considering the importance of the anal cushions for continence and the sensitivity of the terminal

Table 24.1. Theories on etiopathogenesis of hemorrhoidal disease

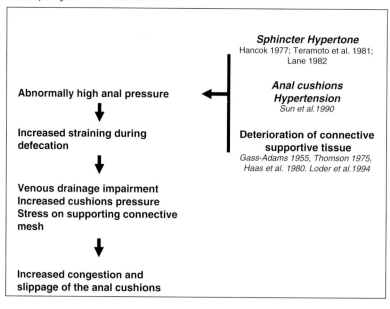

rectal mucosa [17, 29, 30, 31, 32]. However, the most negative outcome after traditional hemorrhoidectomy is the long-lasting intense postoperative pain.

Technique

Transanal hemorrhoidal dearterialization is a nonexcisional surgical method that consists of localization of the terminal branches of the superior rectal artery using a Doppler, and the consequent surgical ligation of those branches. In order to perform this technique, in 1999 I devised; with the collaboration of C. Tagariello, MD, a new instrument named THD[1], a specifically designed proctoscope with a slot into which can fit an apposite Doppler probe. Distally to the Doppler probe there is an operative window that allows the application of the stitches to the rectal mucosa (Fig. 24.1). The tip of the needle holder is inserted inside a pivot in the proctoscope that allows the needle to have always the same precise trajectory

(Fig. 24.2). The proctoscope is illuminated by a light cable inserted through its handle.

The Doppler is used to localize the terminal branches of the superior rectal artery 1–2 cm above the the internal cushions. After complete insertion into the patient's anus, the proctoscope is gently rotated around the rectal circumference in order to locate an audible pulsating arterial signal that confirms that the Doppler transducer is directly above the artery. There are six terminal branches of the superior rectal artery, consistently located at odd hour positions (1, 3, 5, 7, 9, and 11 o'clock; Fig. 24.3). This topography has never been described as a constant, but in clinical practice it is the norm. In several hundred cases of THD performed, I have always been able to locate these branches in the positions described above [45].

After their localization, the arteries are ligated approximately 3 cm above the dentate line with absorbable 2.0 suture mounting a 5/8 short round needle, with a "figure-of-eight" stitch. The knot is tied outside the proctoscope and laid down using a knot pusher. Confirmation of the vessel ligation is performed by repeat Doppler measurements.

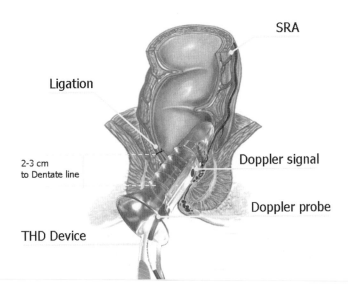

Figure 24.1. THD device description (SRA: superior rectal artery).

[1] THD[tm] by G.F. Medical Division, Correggio, Italy

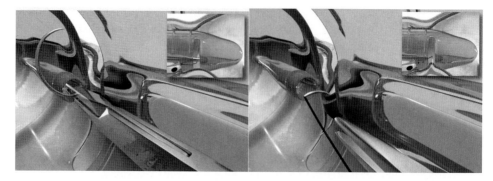

Figure 24.2. Needle rotation inside the device: the needle holder tip is inserted in the pivot and the needle rotates to surround the artery.

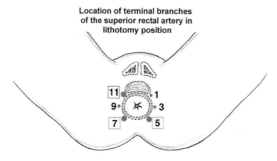

Figure 24.3. Location of the terminal branches of the superior rectal artery.

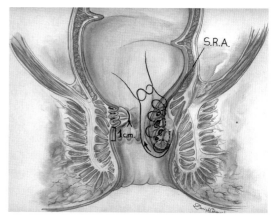

Figure 24.4. Anopexy with running suture (SRA: superior rectal artery).

The reduction or complete absence of the Doppler signal provides evidence of vessel occlusion. This results in decongestion of the hemorrhoidal tissue and alleviation of symptoms. The decreased tension allows for the regeneration of the connective tissue within the cushions. This facilitates the shrinkage of the piles and the reduction of prolapse.

In 2002 we modified the technique described by Morinaga in order to more effectively treat prolapsed hemorrhoids. After the arterial location with the Doppler, a running suture with 3–5 stitches is applied on the prolapsed piles (original technique), in order to surround the prolapsed cushion, being careful that the most distal stitch lies above the dentate line; then the knot is tied at the level of the most cranial stitch in order to lift the prolapse and to occlude the eventual perforating arterial branches (Fig. 24.4). The final outcome of this procedure is a mucosal folding with a fixation to the deeper layers of the rectal wall by the resulting fibrosis. In this way it is possible to obtain a good mucosal pexy and to treat hemorrhoids of third degree with a voluminous prolapse. This technique is to be applied only on those cushions that are prolapsed, and not to be repeated routinely for all six positions described above.

Outcomes

Transanal hemorrhoidal dearterialization is an appropriate technique for day surgery treatment of hemorrhoids, because of the low risk of complication, the low postoperative pain, and therefore the rapid recovery. This procedure can be performed under sedation (Propofol or Midazolam) without local anesthesia. Numerous studies on arterial dearterialization alone, report good results, especially for bleeding second- and third-degree hemorrhoids, with success rates varying from 78% [17] to 100% [50], and with duration of follow-up varying from 4 to 26 months (Table 24.2) [17, 46, 47, 48, 49, 50, 51, 52, 53, 54, 55, 56].

There is only one prospective randomized study in the literature that compares conventional excisional surgery (closed hemorrhoidectomy) with hemorrhoidal dearterialization: it reports an evident advantage of the second method in terms of the use of pain-relieving drugs, with no difference in terms of efficacy at one-year follow-up [57].

Our study is the one with the longest follow-up, and confirms that this technique is safe, effective, and an ideal day surgery procedure for symptomatic hemorrhoids.

Since this method is nonexcisional, the anatomy of the terminal part of the GI tract is fully respected, and consequently so is the physiological function of anal cushions for continence and

of the distal part of the rectum for sensitivity [17,18, 29, 30, 31, 32, 33, 34, 35].

The procedure of Doppler-guided dearterialization as originally described by Morinaga [16], combined with the previously described nonexcisional mucosal pexy, acts on the two previously mentioned components of the pathophysiology of hemorrhoidal disease. This approach has led to an early success rate of 96.7% for bleeding and 95.8% for prolapse in our series of patients. The long-term results at a mean follow-up of 46 months show a success rate of 92.5% for bleeding and 92% for prolapse (Table 24.3).

Overall, in our series, the morbidity from the procedure is low at only 6.4% (Table 24.4). The complications were managed successfully in all cases, with only one patient requiring further surgery for hemorrhage. This is not unsurprising, as the procedure does not depend upon tissue destruction or removal, which can lead to significant postoperative complications. Our outcomes are not significantly different from the complication rate reported in the literature for the dearterialization without anopexy (Table 24.5). For the same reason, transanal dearterialization causes little discomfort. Indeed, over half the patients reported no pain (Table 24.6),

Table 24.2. Results in the literature

Author	N.	Goligher	Follow-up (months)	Success rate	
Morinaga et al. (1995)	113	n.s.	5–12	96%	78%
Menjes et al. (2000)	1415	n.s.	5–24 (1241)	93.2%	
Sohn et al. (2001)	60	II 33%, III 45%, IV 22%		88%	92%
Arnold et al. (2002)	105	II:17%; III:74% IV 9%		89.6%	
Shelygin et al. (2003)	102	III–IV	12 (69 Pt)	82.6%	
Charua Guindic et al. (2004)	49	II: 40;III:9	4	100%	
Lienert et al. (2004)	248		1,5	87.7%	
Infantino et al. (2005)	86	II: 24; III:62	4–26	90%	90%
Felice et al. (2005)	68		11	91%	94%
Ramirez et al. (2005)	36	III–IV	12	78.5%	
Greenberg et al. (2006)	100	II–III	6	94%	
Sheyer et al. (2006)	308	II:89; III:192; IV:26		95.2%	84.4%

II: second-degree hemorrhoids
III: third-degree hemorrhoids
IV: fourth-degree hemorrhoids

Table 24.3. Results (personal series)

SHORT-TERM RESULTS		
330 patients (follow-up: 1 month)		
	BLEEDING: n = 212 (G II:144, G III: 70, G IV:8)	PROLAPSE: n = 192 (G III: 162, G IV: 30)
Resolved	204 (96.7%)	184 (95.8%)
Persisted	8 (3.3%) (G II: 4, G III: 3, G IV: 1)	8 (4.2%) (G III: 3, G IV: 5)
LONG-TERM RESULTS		
219 patients (mean follow-up: 46 months, range 22–79)		
	BLEEDING: n = 142 (G II: 100, G III: 36, G IV: 6)	PROLAPSE: n = 119 (G III: 104, G IV: 15)
Resolved	132 (92.5%)	110 (92%)
Relapsed	10 (7.5%) (G II: 7, G III: 2, G IV: 1)	9 (8%) (G III: 5, G IV: 4)

Table 24.4. Postoperative complications

Bleeding	7; 4 immediate 3 delayed (1 reoperation)
Submucosal hematoma	4
Fissure	2
Thrombosed pile	5
Urinary retention	2
Needle rupture	2
Hematuria	1
TOTAL	23

Table 24.5. Complications in the literature for dearterialization without anopexy

Author	N. Pt.	Complications				
		Thrombosis	Pain	Bleeding	Anal Fissures	Other
Morinaga (1995)	113		6 (5%)	13(12%) (Blood On Stools)		
Sohn (2001)	60	4(7%)	5 (8%)	0	1(2%)	
Bursics	30				3 (10%)	
Infantino	86	1(1.2%)				Urinary retention: 1(1.2%)
Arnold	105	3%			2%	Fistula: 1%
Felice	68	2(3%)		1(1.5%)		
Sheyer	308	9 (2.9%)		3 (1%)	4 (1.3%)	Urinary retention: 4 (1.3%) Fistula: 1 (0.3%)

Table 24.6. Postoperative pain (VAS)

Postoperative pain	N. of patients	
VAS 0	150	
VAS <2	117	
VAS 2–5	35	
VAS 5–8	19	
VAS >8	9	
TOTAL	330	Mean VAS: 1.32

Table 24.7. Analgesia (ketoralac 10 mg tds) requirement

None	186
Up to 2 days	128
Up to 7 days	16
TOTAL	330

and very few required more than two days of analgesia (Table 24.7).

Conclusions

Transanal dearterialization is an effective and safe technique that has excellent results, especially for second- and third-degree hemorrhoids. Furthermore, the hemorrhoidal symptoms of bleeding and prolapse can be successfully treated with relatively few and minor complications and minor postoperative pain. Multicentric studies of comparison with other surgical techniques are necessary to confirm these outcomes.

References

1. Breasted J.H. The Edwin Smith surgical papyrus. Chicago, 1930.
2. Hippocrates. On haemorrhoids:2.
3. Allingham W. Diseases of the rectum (fistula, haemorrhoids, painful ulcer, stricture, prolapsus, and other diseases of the rectum: their diagnosis and treatment). J. and A. Churchill, London, 1871.
4. Whithead W. The surgical treatment of haemorrhoids. Br Med J 1882;1:148–50.
5. Milligan ETC, Morgan CN, Jones LE, Officer R. Surgical anatomy of the anal canal and the operative treatment of haemorrhoids. Lancet 1937;ii:1119–12.
6. Ferguson JA, Heaton JR. Closed hemorrhoidectomy. Dis Colon Rectum 1959;2:176–179.
7. Blaisdell PC. Office ligation of internal hemorrhoids. Am J Surg 1958;96:401–4.
8. Barron J. Office ligation of internal hemorrhoids. Am J Surg 1963;105:563–70.
9. Neiger A. Hemorrhoids in everyday praxis. Proctology 1979;2:22–4.
10. Morgan J. Varicose state of saphenous haemorrhoids treated succesfully by the injection of tincture of persulphate of iron. Medical Press Circular 1869;29–30.
11. Chew SS, Marshall L, Kalish L, Tham J, Grieve DA, Douglas PR, Newstead GL. Short-term and long-term results of combined sclerotherapy and rubber band ligation of hemorrhoids and mucosal prolapse. Dis Colon Rectum. 2003;46:1232–7.
12. Shanmugam V, Thaha M, Rabindranath K, Campbell K, Steele R, Loudon M. Rubber band ligation versus excisional hemorrhoidectomy for hemorrhoids. Cochrane Database Syst Rev 2005 Jul 20;CD005034.
13. Savioz D, Roche B, Glauser T, Dobrinov A, Ludwig C, Marti MC. Rubber band ligation of hemorrhoids: relapse as a function of time. Int J Colorectal Dis 1998;13:154–6.
14. Iyer VS, Shrier I, Gordon PH. Long-term outcome of rubber band ligation for symptomatic primary and recurrent internal hemorrhoids. Dis Colon Rectum 2004;47:1364–70.
15. Longo A. Treatment of hemorrhoids disease by reduction of mucosa and hemorrhoidal prolapse with a circular suturing device: a new procedure. 6th world congress of endoscopic surgery. Rome, Manduzzi 1998:777–784.
16. Morinaga K, Hacuda K, Ikeda T. A novel therapy for internal hemorrhoids: Ligation of the hemorrhoidal artery with a newly devised instrument in conjunction with Doppler flow meter. Am J Gastroenterol 1995;90(4):610–613.
17. Thomson WHF. The nature of hemorrhoids. Br J Surg 1975;62:542–552.
18. Thomson WHF. The anatomy and nature of piles. In: Kaufman HD (ed). The hemorrhoids syndrome. Tunbridge Wells, Kent, England, Abacus Press, 1981:15–33.
19. Thulesis Ø, Gjöres JE. Arteriovenous anastomosis in the anal region with reference to the pathogenesis and treatment of hemorrhoids. Acta Chir Scand 1973;139:476–478.
20. Haas PA, Fox TA, Haas GP. The pathogenesis of hemorrhoids. Dis Colon Rectum 1984;27:442–450
21. Stelzner F, Staubesand J, Machleidt H. Das Corpus Cavernosum Recti—die Grundlage der inneren Hämorrhoiden. Langenbecks Arch Klein Chir 1962;299:302–312.
22. Widmer O. Die Rectalarterien des Menschen. Z Anat Entwicklungsgesch 1955;118:398–416.
23. Patricio J, Bernades A, Nuno D et al. Surgical anatomy of the arterial blood supply of the human rectum. Surg Radiol Anat 1988;10:71–5.
24. Sun WM, Read NW, Shorthouse AJ. Hypertensive anal cushions as a cause of high anal canal pressures in patients with haemorrhoids. Br J Surg 1990;77:458–62.
25. Shafik A, Mostafa H. Study of the arterial pattern of the rectum and its clinical application. Acta Anat 1996;157:80–6.

26. Aigner F, Bodner G, Conrad F, Mbaka G, Kreczy A, Fritsch H. The superior rectal artery and its branching pattern with regard to its clinical influence on ligation techniques for internal hemorrhoids. Am J Surg 2004;187:102–108.

27. Stelzner F, Fleischhauer F, Holstein AF. Die Bedeutung des Sphincter internus für die Analkontinenz. Langenbecks Arch Klein Chir 1966;314:132–136.

28. Hansen HH. Die Bedeutung des M. canalis ani für die Kontinenz und anorectale Erkrankungen. Langenbecks Arch Chir 1976;341:23–37.

29. Gibbons CP, Trowbridge EA, Bannister JJ, Read NW. The role of the anal cushions in maintaining continence. Lancet 1986;i:886–887.

30. Lestar B, Penninckx F, Rigauts H, Kerremans R. The internal anal sphincter cannot close the anal canal completely. Int J Colorectal Dis 1992;7:159–161.

31. Penninckx F, Lestar B, Kerremans R. The internal anal sphincter: mechanisms of control and its role in maintaining anal continence. Baill Clin Gastroenterol 1992;6(1):193–214.

32. Holzheimer RG. Hemorrhoidectomy: indications and risks. Eur J Med Res 2004;9:18–36.

33. American Gastroenterological Association. Technical review on the diagnosis and treatment of hemorrhoids. Gastroenterology 2004;126:1463–1473.

34. Gass OC, Adams J. Hemorrhoids: etiology and pathology. Am J Surg 1950;79:40–43.

35. Loder PB, Kamm MA, Nicholls RJ. Haemorrhoids: pathology, pathophysiology and aetiology. Br J Surg 1994;81:946–954.

36. Stelzner F. Die Haemorroiden und andere Krankheit des Corpus cavernosum recti und des Analkanals. Dtsch Med Wochenschr 1963;88:689–96.

37. Lane RHS. Measurement of anal pressure in patients with haemorrhoids. Schweiz Rundsch Med Prax 1982;71:112–5.

38. Teramoto T, Parks AG, Swash M. Hypertrophy of the external anal sphincter in haemorrhoids: a histometric study. Gut 1981;22(1):45–8.

39. Wldron DJ, Kumar D, Hallan RI, Williams NS. Prolonged ambulant assessment of anorectal function in patients with prolapsing hemorrhoids. Dis Colon Rectum 1989;32:968–74.

40. Sun WM, Peck RJ, Shorthouse AJ, Read NW. Haemorrhoids are associated not with hypertrophy of the internal sphincter, but with hypertension of the anal cushions. Br J Surg 1992;78:592–4.

41. Hancock BD. Internal sphincter and the nature of haemorrhoids. Gut 1977;18:651–656.

42. Shafik A. The pathogenesis of hemorrhoids and their treatment by anorectal bandotomy. J Clin Gastroenterol 1984;6:129–137.

43. Read NW, Harford WV, Schmulen AC et al. A clinical study of patients with faecal incontinence and diarrhea. Gastroenterology 1979;76:747–56.

44. Read MG, Read NW, Haynes WG, Donnelly TC, Johnson AG. A prospective study of the effect of haemorrhoidectomy on sphincter function and faecal continence. Br J Surg 1982;69:396–398.

45. Dal Monte PP. Doppler-guided hemorrhoidal artery ligation. Tech Coloproctol 2006 Oct;10(3):262; discussion 263.

46. Meintjes D. Doppler-guided hemorrhoidal artery ligation (HAL) for the treatment of hemorrhoids. Results in 1415 patients. Clin Rep 2000.

47. Sohn N, Aronoff JS, Cohen FS, Weinstein MA. Transanal hemorrhoidal dearterialization is an alternative to operative hemorrhoidectomy. Am J Surg. 2001;182:515–9.

48. Arnold S, Antonietti E, Rollinger G, Scheyer M. Doppler ultrasound assisted hemorrhoid artery ligation. A new therapy in symptomatic hemorrhoids. Chirurg 2002 Mar;73(3):269–73.

49. Shelygin IuA, Titov AIu, Veselov VV, Kanametov MKh. Results of ligature of distal branches of the upper rectal artery in chronic hemorrhoid with the assistance of Doppler ultrasonography. Khirurgiia (Mosk) 2003;(1):39–44.

50. Charua Guindic L, Fonseca Munoz E, Garcia Perez NJ, Osorio Hernandez RM, Navarrete Cruces T, Avendano Espinosa O, Guerra Melgar LR. Hemorrhoidal dearterialization guided by Doppler. A surgical alternative in hemorrhoidal disease management. Rev Gastroenterol Mex. 2004;69:83–7.

51. Lienert M, Ulrich B. Doppler-guided ligation of the hemorrhoidal arteries. Report of experiences with 248 patients. Dtsch Med Wochenschr 2004;129:947–50.

52. Infantino A, Amadio L, Bellomo R, Tonizzo CA, Romano G, Bianco F, Salafia C, Altomare D, Dal Monte PP, Saragò M, Tagariello C. Doppler-guided transanal hemorrhoidal dearterialisation is a valid treatment option for II- and III-degree hemorrhoidal disease. Proceedings of the second joint meeting, European council of coloproctology, September 15–17, 2005, Bologna, Italy. Monduzzi Editore, 2006.

53. Ramirez JM, Aguilella V, Elia M, Gracia JA, Martinez M. D Doppler-guided hemorrhoidal artery ligation in the management of symptomatic hemorrhoids. Rev Esp Enferm Dig 2005;97:97–103.

54. Greenberg R, Karin E, Avital S, Skornick Y, Werbin N. First 100 cases with Doppler-guided hemorrhoidal artery ligation. Dis Colon Rectum 2006 Apr;49(4):485–9.

55. Scheyer M, Antonietti E, Rollinger G, Mall H, Arnold S. Doppler-guided hemorrhoidal artery ligation. Am J Surg. 2006 Jan;191(1):89–93.

56. Bursics A, Morvay K, Kupcsulik P, Flautner L. Comparison of early and 1-year follow-up results of conventional hemorrhoidectomy and hemorrhoid artery ligation: a randomized study. Int J Colorectal Dis. 2004;1:176–80.

57. Dal Monte PP, Tagariello C, Giordano P, Cudazzo E, Shafi A, Sarago M, Franzini M. Transanal hemorrhoidal dearterialisation: nonexcisonal surgery for the treatment of haemorrhoidal disease. Tech Coloproctol 2007;4:333–339.

25 Semiclosed Hemorrhoidectomy

Fidel Ruiz-Healy, Abel Morales-Diaz, and Javier H. Figueroa-Becerra

---

Introduction

The semiclosed hemorrhoidectomy is a modification of the classic ligation and excision technique. It was first described in 1971 as the Ruiz-Moreno technique, by other authors [1]. In 1973, Reis Neto described a variant of this procedure with good results [2]. Several publications referring to semiclosed technique have followed [3, 4, 5, 6, 7, 8]. Many surgeons in Latin America [9] and Japan [10] prefer the semiclosed hemorrhoidectomy.

Operative Technique

Preoperative Management

Routine preoperative workup includes laboratory tests (complete blood count, coagulation profile, blood glucose, urinalysis, serological investigation of hepatitis C, HIV, and amebiasis) as well as evaluations by the internal medicine and anesthesia practitioners. The patient is kept NPO after midnight and is usually admitted the morning of surgery. Evacuating suppositories are administered on admission and two hours before surgery.

Position of Patient

The prone position is used, with two pillows raising the pelvic area. No tapes are applied to separate the buttocks. We do not shave the perianal area. The area is prepped with a colorless, nonirritant antiseptic solution.

Anesthesia

Lumbar epidural analgesia is administered by an anesthesiologist. The catheter is left in place during the surgical procedure and removed upon termination of the operation.

Insertion of Operative Speculum

A Pratt bivalve speculum is lubricated with an aqueous jelly lubricant and introduced into the lower rectum. Physiologic solution with an aspirator is used to wash the anal canal and lower rectum.

Anchorage Stitch in Lower Mucosa

Using a Fansler or Pratt bivalve speculum, we localize the hemorrhoidal complex. With a long Russian forceps, we grasp the redundant rectal mucosa well above the internal hemorrhoidal tissue. Using slight traction we apply a deep anchoring stitch, including the muscle layer, using a 4-0 or 5-0 monofilament synthetic absorbable surgical suture (Fig. 25.1, reproduced from Ruiz Moreno F. Hemorrhoidectomy—how I do it: semiclosed technique. Dis Colon Rectum 1977;20:177–182. With kind permission of Lippincott Williams & Wilkins).

I. Khubchandani et al. (eds.), *Surgical Treatment of Hemorrhoids*, DOI 10.1007/978-1-84800-314-9_25,
© Springer-Verlag London Limited 2009

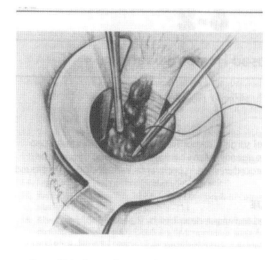

Figure 25.1. Deep anchoring stitch including muscle layer.

1977;20:177–182. With kind permission of Lippincott Williams & Wilkins).

Dissection of Hemorrhoidal Tissue

With a fine Metzenbaum scissors we dissect and separate the hemorrhoidal complex from the muscle layers. The subcutaneous external sphincter muscle, internal anal sphincter, and the circular muscle fibers of the lower rectum are identified and left intact. Dissection is carried down to the anchoring stitch. To minimize trauma, suction is used instead of gauze sponges. Small bleeding vessels are clamped and fulgurated. Larger vessels are sutured with a 4-0 monofilament synthetic absorbable surgical suture (Fig. 25.2).

Incision Around the Hemorrhoidal Tissue

With a small scalpel, a long and narrow inverted drop-form incision is created by starting at the site of the anchorage stitch, and continuing up through the lower rectum, the anal canal, and the perianal skin, going around the hemorrhoidal mass and back down to the starting point. The depth of the incision reaches the mucosa and submucosa, leaving intact the circular muscle layer (Fig. 25.2, reproduced from Ruiz Moreno F. Hemorrhoidectomy—how I do it: semiclosed technique. Dis Colon Rectum

Semiclosing the Wound

With the same anchored suture, we close both ends of open mucosa with a continuous or locking suture up to the dentate line. In order to obtain wound integrity, the suture is to be wide and deep, including mucosa, submucosa, and muscle (Fig. 25.3, reproduced from Ruiz Moreno F. Hemorrhoidectomy—how I do it: semiclosed technique. Dis Colon Rectum 1977;20:177–182. With kind permission of Lippincott Williams & Wilkins). From this point, only one border is sutured in a continuous or locking manner and approximating

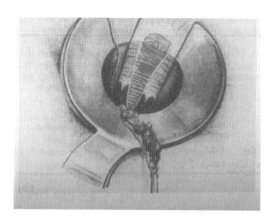

Figure 25.2. Incision and dissection of hemorrhoidol tissue.

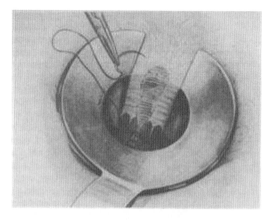

Figure 25.3. Suture closing both ends of mucosa up to dentate line.

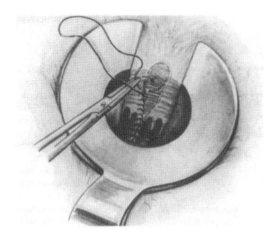

Figure 25.4. Suture of one border, starting at denate line.

the border to the middle of the open wound, up to
the perianal skin (Fig. 25.4, reproduced from Ruiz
Moreno F. Hemorrhoidectomy—how I do it: semiclosed   technique.   Dis   Colon   Rectum
1977;20:177–182. With kind permission of Lippincott Williams & Wilkins).

The other border of the wound is sutured in the
same way as the first side. Continuous or locking sutures are done without tension. The open
wound is reduced, producing a narrow semiclosed
wound (Fig. 25.5, reproduced from Ruiz Moreno
F. Hemorrhoidectomy—how I do it: semiclosed
technique. Dis Colon Rectum 1977;20:177–182.
With kind permission of Lippincott Williams &
Wilkins).

Removal of Other Hemorrhoidal Tissues

The speculum is removed, lubricated, and placed
where another hemorrhoidal complex is localized.
The same procedure as described above is performed. The size of the wound depends on the
size of the hemorrhoidal complex. Three to six
incisions are done. It is very important to leave
approximately 1 cm bridges with good circulation between wounds (Fig. 25.6, reproduced from
Ruiz Moreno F. hemorrhoidectomy—how I do
it: semiclosed technique. Dis Colon Rectum
1977;20:177–182. With kind permission of
Lippincott Williams & Wilkins).

Finishing Procedures

With a Pratt bivalve speculum, saline solution
is used to wash the anorectal area. With a
Mayo speculum, we check for bleeding sites.
We usually do not leave any packing within
the rectum.

Postoperative Management

Our patients routinely pass through the recovery room. Intravenous fluid restriction during
the transoperative and immediate postoperative

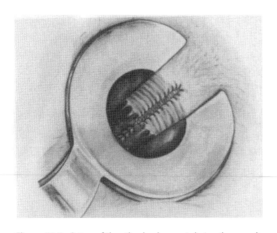

Figure 25.5. Suture of the other border, semi-closing the wound.

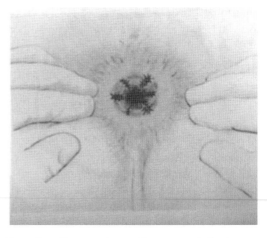

Figure 25.6. Three to six incisions. Mucocutaneous bridges between wounds.

period helps keep bladder catheterization to a minimum. Analgesics are administered as needed by oral, IM, or IV route. A high-fiber diet is given 6–8 h after surgical intervention. Sitz baths are initiated early the next morning, and the patient is usually discharged from the hospital 24 h postop. Patients are followed up in the office approximately three times during the first week, twice during the second and third weeks, and once during the fourth week. Upon final surgical discharge, patients are seen after the first month, then after six months, and later, once a year.

Results

There are few comparative studies between semiclosed hemorrhoidectomy and other techniques. Catan and Catan reviewed their personal experience in 100 hemorrhoidectomies, comparing closed and semiclosed techniques, favoring the semiclosed hemorrhoidectomy [4]. In a randomized trial of 300 patients, comparing open and semi-open technique, Reis Neto et al. found the semi-open technique superior to the open technique [5]. Mikuni et al., in a prospective randomized trial of 34 patients, comparing open and semiclosed hemorrhoidectomy, found small differences between the techniques [10]. Pescatori, in a 12-patient report, performing a two-quadrant semiclosed hemorrhoidectomy, found good results with regard to bleeding rate, healing process, operative time, and postoperative pain [11].

Postoperative Pain

Catan and Catan reported that pain was present in all patients operated on with the closed technique, and significant in a great number of patients operated on with the semiclosed technique [4].

Reis Neto found that patients operated on with the semi-open technique suffered less intense pain that those who had had the open technique, both during the immediate postoperative hospitalization, and in the later ambulatory phase [5].

Mikuni et al. reported that both groups, having each received the same amount of pain medication, reported same pain scores during the first and third postoperative days as well as after the second week. A higher pain score is reported at one week (P = 0.018) and two weeks (P = 0.066) in patients operated on with the semiclosed technique [10]. Pescatori, using the semiclosed technique, found that the mean postoperative pain after 12 h, measured from 1 to 10 on a visual analogue scale, was 4.4 (SEM = 1.4) [11].

Immediate Postoperative Complications

Catan and Catan reported 8% urinary retention after the closed hemorrhoidectomy and none after the semiclosed hemorrhoidectomy [4]. Reis Neto found 11.3% urinary retention with the open technique and 4% with the semi-open technique, as well as immediate hemorrhage in one patient (0.6%) after the open technique [5].

Late Postoperative Complications

Reis Neto reported residual skin tags of 7.3% using the open technique versus 0.6% using the semi-open technique [5]. Catan and Catan found a 12% occurrence of postoperative stenosis using the closed technique versus 2% using the semiclosed technique [4]. Late hemorrhage, abscess, and fistula formation were not reported by any of the four authors.

Healing Time

Catan and Catan observed an average of 10 days healing time after the closed technique and 18 days after the semiclosed technique [4]. Reis Neto reported an average of 25.2 days after the open hemorrhoidectomy and 12.4 days after the semi-open hemorrhoidectomy [5]. Pescatori found that all wounds were healed within 3 weeks after semiclosed hemorrhoidectomy [11].

Conclusions

Hemorrhoidectomy by the semiclosed technique is an excellent option in the management of mixed hemorrhoidal disease with large mucocutaneous components. Pain is moderate, recovery is rapid, complications are few, and the long-term results are very good [7].

References

1. Galvan ES, Villagi Leyva JC, Borracer G. Hemorroidectomia. Técnica de Ruiz Moreno. Pren Med Argent 1971;58:953–958.
2. 10. Reis Neto JA. Hemorroidectomia semi-fechada. Actas del 5° Congreso Argentino e Internacional de Proctologia. Mar de Plata, Argentina, 1973, Tomo II:94.
3. Ruiz Moreno F. Hemorrhoidectomy—how I do it: semiclosed technique. Dis Colon Rectum 1977; 20:177–182.
4. Catan LB, Catan F. Hemorroidectomia—Experiencia adquirida em dados comparatives entre duas técnicas operatorias. Rev Bras Colo-Proct 1985;5:155–160.
5. Reis Neto JA, Quilici FA, Cordeiro F, Reis JA Jr. Open versus semi-open hemorrhoidectomy. A random trial. Int Surg 1992;77:84–90.
6. Ruiz Moreno F, Ruiz Healy F. Hemorroidectomia. Técnica semicerrada. Cirug y Cirujan 1997;45:161–165.
7. Ruiz-Healy F, Morales-Diaz A. Semiclosed hemorrhoidectomy. In: J.A. Reis Neto (ed). New trends in coloproctology, 1st ed. Rio de Janeiro, Livraria e Editora RevinteR, 2000:191–196.
8. Reis Neto JA, Reis JA Jr, Kagohara O, Simoes Neto J. Semi-open hemorrhoidectomy. Tech Coloproctol 2005;9:159–161.
9. Saravia-Leao PE. Hemorróidas. Fatos e Ficcoes, 1st ed. Fortaleza-Ceará, Ediciones EUFC, 1988.
10. Mikuni N, Oya M, Komatsu J, Yamana T. A prospective randomized comparison between an open hemorrhoidectomy and a semiclosed (semi-open) hemorrhoidectomy. Surg Today 2002;32:40–47.
11. Pescatori M. Two-quadrant semiclosed hemorrhoidectomy. Tech Coloproctol 2002;6:105–108.

26 Hemorrhoidectomy Using the Ligasure™ Vessel Sealing System

S. Roka, A. Salat, and B. Teleky

Immediate complications of surgical procedures for the treatment of hemorrhoids are postoperative pain and bleeding [1]. Bleeding after hemorrhoidectomy is rare but often requires a surgical procedure or even administration of blood units. Hemorrhoidectomy according to Milligan-Morgan or Ferguson is nowadays carried out with conventional diathermy to reduce intraoperative and postoperative blood loss. A number of new hemostatic devices have been developed in the past decade, that have also been tested for hemorrhoidectomy [2]. One of them is the Ligasure™ Vessel Sealing System (LS).

The system consists of a generator and a choice of nine different instruments [2]. Only two of these instruments are used for hemorrhoidectomy (Ligasure™ Max handset, Ligasure™ Precise). Both of them are shaped like a surgical clamp with different angles of deflection and work as a bipolar clamp. The generator produces a high-current, low-voltage pulsed output. The current compares to at least four times the current and 5–20% of the voltage produced by a standard electrosurgery generator. Because of a feedback mechanism, changes in the tissue are sensed 200 times per second, and voltage and current are adapted accordingly. The completion of the sealing process is indicated by an acoustic signal. The device effects a permanent seal by melting collagen and elastin in the vessel walls, thereby reforming a permanent, plastic-like seal. Vessel sealing doesn't need to rely on the formation of a proximal thrombus. The devices are suitable for sealing vessels up to 7 mm in diameter. Because of the design of the instruments, lateral thermal spread is diminished (1–2 mm) and tissue temperature does not exceed 100° Celsius.

Indications for LS in Hemorrhoidectomy

The LS device helps to achieve hemostasis. The principle of the surgical procedure is the same as in open or closed hemorrhoidectomy. Therefore the indications are the same and comprise stage III and IV hemorrhoids.

Surgical Procedure

An anal retractor is introduced to visualize the surgical field. The hemorrhoidal complex is grasped by Allis clamps. It is important to elevate the skin to be able to see the junction between the hemorrhoid and the perianal skin (the site where the incision should be made (Fig. 26.1). Now the LS device can be applied. Not too much tissue should be pulled into the jaws of the device, to reduce damage to the internal anal sphincter. To reduce the risk of postoperative bleeding, the vascular pedicle of the hemorrhoids can be sealed twice (Fig. 26.2).

I. Khubchandani et al. (eds.), *Surgical Treatment of Hemorrhoids*, DOI 10.1007/978-1-84800-314-9_26,
© Springer-Verlag London Limited 2009

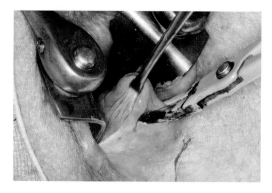

Figure 26.1 Start of preparation between haemorrhoid and perianal skin.

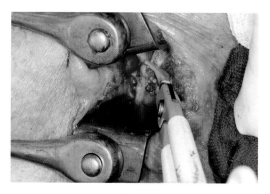

Figure 26.2 Sealing of the vascular pedicle using the LigaSure™ device.

A different method has been described involving a submucosal dissection [3] before applying the LS device. By conventional dissection the submucous plane is demonstrated. Thereby the internal anal sphincter can be identified to avoid damage. The LS device is only applied to the mucosa and vascular pedicle.

Trials of LS Hemorrhoidectomy

The surgical technique using LS for hemorrhoidectomy has been evaluated in several prospective randomized studies (Table 26.1). Most of these compared hemorrhoidectomy using the LS device to conventional closed or open

hemorrhoidectomy using conventional diathermy. There have also been studies comparing LS with hemorrhoidectomy using the harmonic scalpel or stapled hemorrhoidectomy.

Operative Time

Using LS reduced the time of the surgical procedure in all studies comparing LS to conventional open or closed hemorrhoidectomy. The average time for the procedure using LS varies considerably between the different studies (5.1–23 min). Only a minority of these studies state the surgical time for each hemorrhoid bundle. One study showed LS to be more time efficient, compared to hemorrhoidectomy using the harmonic scalpel [4]. Two studies comparing LS to stapled hemorrhoidectomy show conflicting results [5, 6].

Postoperative Pain and Use of Pain Medication

In all studies a visual analog scale was used to assess postoperative pain.

Four studies comparing LS to conventional hemorrhoidectomy used a standardized pain medication for all patients. In three of these studies [7, 8, 9] postoperative pain was significantly less after hemorrhoidectomy using LS; the fourth [10] showed a benefit for LS as well, but it was not statistically significant.

In the other studies pain medication was not standardized [11, 12, 3]. In general, less pain medication was used for patients after LS than conventional hemorrhoidectomy. Most of these studies also showed that there was less postoperative pain after LS hemorrhoidectomy. However, this difference was only significant in one study [3].

Two studies comparing LS to stapled hemorrhoidectomy found conflicting results. In the study by Kraemer et al. [6] use of pain medication and postoperative pain were less for patients after

Table 26.1 Studies comparing hemorrhoidectomy using LigaSure with other techniques.

study	n	technique	surgical time (min)	postoperative pain		postoperative complications (%)					hospital stay	return to work
				pain medication	pain VAS	bleeding	urinary retention	incontinence	stenosis	delayed healing/fissure		
Palazzo [11]	18	LS	5.1*	less in favor of Ligasure*	5.2	0 (0)		0 (0)	0 (0)			
	16	DT	9.2*		4.6	3 (12.7)		0 (0)	0 (0)			
Muzi [7]	125	LS	11.5*	standardized	1.5*	1 (0.8)		0 (0)	1 (0.8)		8.2 h	
	125	DT	20*		3.3*	2 (1.6)		0 (0)	1 (0.8)		10.3 h	
Franklin [8]	17	LS	6*	less in favor of LS *				0 (0)				
	17	DT	11*					0 (0)				
Jayne [9]	20	LS	10*	standardized	5	1 (5)	1 (5)	0 (0)		1 (5)	earlier discharge in favor of LS	
	20	DT	20*		7	1 (5)	0 (0)	0 (0)		1 (5)		
Pattana-Arun [12]	23	LS	21.7*	no difference		0 (0)	1 (4.3)			5 (21.7)		
	22	DT	35.7*			0 (0)	2 8.6			4 (18.2)		
Wang [3]	42	LS	11.5*	less in favor of LS	5.1*	1 (2.4)	2 (4.8)	0 (0)	1 (2.4)	no difference	2.2 d	8.8 d*
	42	DT	34.2*		7.2*	1 (2.4)	5 (11.9)	1 (2.4)	2 (4.8)		2.9 d	13.7 d*
Basdanis [5]	50	STH	15*	less in favor of STH	3*	3 (6)		1 (2)			1.6 d	6.8 d*
	45	LS	13*		6*	1 (2.9)		2 (5.8)			2.1 d	9.8 d*
Kwok [4]	24	LS	11*	less in favor of LS *	2.6*	1 (4.2)	3 (12.5)	0 (0)	0 (0)	0 (0)	2 d	
	25	HS	18*		4.8*	2 (8)	4 (16)	1 (4)	0 (0)	0 (0)	3 d	
Chung [10]	30	LS	15.0*	standardized	less in favor of LS	1 (3.3)	2 (6.6)				3.2 d	
	31	DT	21.2*			0 (0)	4 (12.9)				3.5 d	
Kraemer [6]	25	LS	23	less in favor of LS	no difference	1 (4)	2 (8)				5.0 d	
	25	STH	20			0 (0)	4 (16)				4.0 d	

* Indicates significant results; LS: LigaSure hemorrhoidectomy, DT: conventional hemorrhoidectomy using diathermy, STH: stapled hemorrhoidectomy, HS: Harmonic Scalpel

LS. The study by Basdanis [5] found the opposite for stapled hemorrhoidectomy. In the study by Kwok et al. [4] use of pain medication and postoperative pain was less in patients after LS hemorrhoidectomy, compared to hemorrhoidectomy using the harmonic scalpel.

Hospital Stay and Return to Work

Different protocols have been obtained in the studies in regard to the management of hemorrhoidectomy towards day-case or inpatient treatment. The postoperative stay after day-case surgery was shorter for LS compared to conventional hemorrhoidectomy in the study by Muzi et al. [7] There was slight but not significant benefit in three studies comparing LS to conventional hemorrhoidectomy as inpatient treatment [9, 3, 10]. There was also no significant difference in studies comparing LS to stapled hemorrhoidectomy [5, 6] or using the harmonic scalpel [4].

Two studies showed a significantly earlier return to work for LS compared to conventionel hemorrhoidectomy [3] and stapled hemorrhoidectomy [5].

Complications

In none of the studies was a difference found in the incidence of postoperative complications. The incidence of postoperative bleeding was lower for LS hemorrhoidectomy in all but two studies [6, 10]. In all but one study [9] the incidence of postoperative urinary retention was lower after LS hemorrhoidectomy. Deterioration of continence or anal stenosis have been rare events in all studies. Delayed healing and postoperative anal fissure have been defined differently in most studies. Differences between studies are therefore considerable, but no difference was seen in favor of any method of hemorrhoidectomy.

Conclusion

The main complications after conventional hemorrhoidectomy (open or closed) are postoperative pain, bleeding, urinary retention, deterioration of continence, and anal stenosis. To overcome these problems, a variety of different surgical procedures have been described, and the technique of hemorrhoidectomy has been modified, especially after the introduction of new hemostatic devices like the Ligasure^{TM} Vessel Sealing System.

The available studies show that using the Ligasure^{TM} Vessel Sealing System for hemorrhoidectomy is safe. Postoperative complications are the same as after conventional hemorrhoidectomy and there is no difference in the incidence of postoperative complications. The operative time is reduced and there seems to be a positive influence on postopeative pain compared to some other treatment options.

Open or closed conventional hemorrhoidectomy is a standardized procedure that can be performed with minimal technical and monetary efforts. Advocates of hemostatic devices argue that the higher expenses are offset by a shorter time for surgery, reduced use of postoperative pain medication, a shorter hospital stay, and an earlier return to work. However, these variables depend on individual treatment protocols and local habits.

References

1. Sardinha TC, Corman ML. Hemorrhoids. Surg Clin North Am 2002;82(6):1153–67, vi.
2. Fleshman J. Advanced technology in the management of hemorrhoids: stapling, laser, harmonic scalpel, and Liga-Sure. J Gastrointest Surg 2002;6(3):299–301.
3. Wang JY, Lu CY, Tsai HL, Chen FM, Huang CJ, Huang YS, Huang TJ, Hsieh JS. Randomized controlled trial of Liga-Sure with submucosal dissection versus Ferguson hemorrhoidectomy for prolapsed hemorrhoids. World J Surg 2006;30(3):462–6.
4. Kwok SY, Chung CC, Tsui KK, Li MK. A double-blind, randomized trial comparing Ligasure and Harmonic Scalpel hemorrhoidectomy. Dis Colon Rectum 2005;48(2):344–8.
5. Basdanis G, Papadopoulos VN, Michalopoulos A, Apostolidis S, Harlaftis N. Randomized clinical trial of stapled

hemorrhoidectomy vs. open with LigaSure for prolapsed piles. Surg Endosc 2005;19(2):235–9.

6. Kraemer M, Parulava T, Roblick M, Duschka L, Muller-Lobeck H. (2005) Prospective, randomized study: proximate PPH stapler vs. LigaSure for hemorrhoidal surgery. Dis Colon Rectum 2005;48(8):1517–22.

7. Muzi MG, Milito G, Nigro C, Cadeddu F, Andreoli F, Amabile D, Farinon AM. Randomized clinical trial of LigaSure and conventional diathermy haemorrhoidectomy. Br J Surg 2007;94(8):937–42.

8. Franklin EJ, Seetharam S, Lowney J, Horgan PG. Randomized, clinical trial of Ligasure vs conventional diathermy in hemorrhoidectomy. Dis Colon Rectum 2003;46(10):1380–3.

9. Jayne DG, Botterill I, Ambrose NS, Brennan TG, Guillou PJ, O'Riordain DS. Randomized clinical trial of LigaSure versus conventional diathermy for day-case haemorrhoidectomy. Br J Surg 2002;89(4):428–32.

10. Chung YC, Wu HJ. Clinical experience of sutureless closed hemorrhoidectomy with LigaSure. Dis Colon Rectum 2003;46(1):87–92.

11. Palazzo FF, Francis DL, Clifton MA. Randomized clinical trial of Ligasure versus open haemorrhoidectomy. Br J Surg 2002;89(2):154–7.

12. Pattana-Arun J, Sooriprasoet N, Sahakijrungruang C, Tantiphlachiva K, Rojanasakul A. Closed vs. LigaSure hemorrhoidectomy: a prospective, randomized clinical trial. J Med Assoc Thai 2006;89(4):453–8.

27 Limited Hemorrhoidectomy

Martin A. Luchtefeld and Irfan Rizvi

Approximately only 10% of patients with symptomatic hemorrhoids have symptoms severe enough to warrant excisional hemorrhoidectomy. This has traditionally been a three-column excision in patients failing nonoperative treatment. In the vast majority of cases such procedures are successfully carried out on an outpatient basis. Hunt et al. [1] have shown that day-case hemorrhoidectomy is feasible in 82% of selected patients and results in a high degree of satisfaction among patients. At our institution we have also been able to achieve similar results based on a standardized protocol that involves perioperative local anesthetic block followed by a standardized regimen of scheduled NSAIDS (Motrin), gabapentin, fiber, and supplemental opiate analgesia. This has served to reduce immediate postoperative pain, facilitate a comfortable first bowel movement, and minimize the incidence of urinary retention by restricting intraoperative fluid administration.

There has been a trend in recent years to resist the traditional surgical approach to hemorrhoids and to do limited (one- or two-quadrant) hemorrhoidectomy. The idea of symptom-based treatment of hemorrhoids is not unique to hemorrhoidectomy. In an early series of hemorrhoidal banding, anywhere from one to three bands were applied to control symptoms [2, 3]. In the series of Wrobleski et al., those who received a single band were as likely to get symptom relief as those who had multiple bands placed [3].

While Khubchandani found no significant difference in complications when comparing a single band to muliple bands [2], there is some evidence in the literature to suggest that a more directed approach to rubber band ligation of hemorrhoidal pedicles may lower the incidence of complications associated with the procedure. Lee et al. [4] have reported an increased risk of discomfort (29% in multiple bandings versus 4.5% in single bandings), vasovagal symptoms (5.2% in multiple bandings versus 0% in single bandings), and urinary symptoms (12.3% in multiple bandings versus 0% in single bandings) in patients presenting for this treatment.

While the majority of patients undergo a three-quadrant hemorrhoidectomy, there has been a shift towards a more directed approach of excising quadrants that dominate or are responsible for patient symptoms. Hayssen et al. [5] reported a comparative study of 115 patients with limited hemorrhoidectomy versus an age-matched and gender-matched control group of 133 patients with three-quadrant hemorrhoidectomy. Twenty-six patients and eighty-nine patients underwent a one- and two-quadrant hemorrhoidectomy, respectively, for symptoms of bleeding, swelling, and protrusion. Significantly more complications were reported in patients undergoing two-quadrant and three-quadrant excision. The most common postoperative complication was urinary retention, occurring in 29% of patients in the two-quadrant group and in 40% of the three-quadrant group. Patients with one-quadrant hemorrhoidectomy experienced urinary retention in less than 5% of the cases (n = 1). Relief of symptoms was

I. Khubchandani et al. (eds.), *Surgical Treatment of Hemorrhoids*, DOI 10.1007/978-1-84800-314-9_27,
© Springer-Verlag London Limited 2009

experienced in over 96% of the patients in all groups. No significant difference in recurrence of symptoms was found between the limited and three-column hemorrhoidectomy groups. Although bleeding, swelling, and protrusion were reported after hemorrhoidectomy, the majority of patients could be successfully treated with observation or conservative measures. Only 1.7% of all patients in the limited hemorrhoidectomy group required an additional procedure (rubber band ligation, n = 2) with mean follow-up of 8 years. No patient in either group required additional excisional hemorrhoidectomy for recurrent symptoms.

Hemorrhoidectomy is susceptible to complications. They include urinary retention, secondary hemorrhage, anal stricture, infection, and impairment of continence. Some 5–10% of patients undergoing day-case hemorrhoidectomy require readmission. Zaheer et al. [6] conducted a study to determine the incidence and risk factors for urinary retention after operations for benign anorectal diseases. They reviewed 1,026 consecutive operations for benign anorectal diseases and reported a 34% rate of urinary retention following hemorrhoidectomy. The number of quadrants excised was an independent risk factor (with four-quadrant excision having a higher odds ratio [3.3; P = 0.0004] compared to three-quadrant excision [2.4; P = 0.003]) along with the amount of morphine used (in our view, itself related to the extent of surgery), and male gender.

Limited symptom-directed hemorrhoidectomy appears to have few drawbacks and potentially can be done with less pain and fewer complications than the traditional hemorrhoidectomy. For patients with limited hemorrhoidal disease, this option should remain a consideration for the surgeon.

References

1. Hunt L, Luck AJ, Rudkin G, Hewett PJ. Day-case haemorrhoidectomy. Br J Surg 1999;86:255–8.
2. Khubchandani IT. A randomized comparison of single and multiple rubber band ligations. Dis Colon Rectum 1983; 26:705.
3. Wrobleski DE, Corman ML, Veidenheimer MC et al. Long-term evaluation of rubber ring ligation in hemorrhoidal disease. Dis Colon Rectum 1980;23:478.
4. Hayssen TK, Luchtefeld MA, Senagore AJ. Limited hemorrhoidectomy: results and long-term follow-up. Dis Colon Rectum 1999;42:909–14; discussion 914–5.
5. Lee HH, Spencer RJ, Beart RW Jr. Multiple hemorrhoidal bandings in a single session. Dis Colon Rectum 1994;37: 37–41.
6. Zaheer S, Reily WT, Pemberton JH, Ilstrup D. Urinary retention after operations for benign anorectal disease. Dis Colon Rectum 1998 Jun;41(6):696–704.

28 Hemorrhoid Therapy for Patients on Medications Altering Coagulation

Jeffrey Albright and H. Randolph Bailey

Symptomatic hemorrhoids represent an extremely common disorder, affecting essentially all age groups. A variety of office and surgical procedures have been developed to treat this condition. A recognized complication of all treatments for hemorrhoids is late bleeding secondary to mucosal ulceration or sloughing of the vascular pedicle. This event usually occurs while the patient is at home and can be life threatening. For this reason, medications that alter normal coagulation are typically discontinued prior to treatment of the symptomatic hemorrhoids if it is deemed safe to do so.

An increasing number of patients are taking medications that alter coagulation. These medications, which include aspirin, nonsteroidal anti-inflammatory drugs (NSAIDs), thienopyridines (clopidogrel and ticlopidine), and warfarin, inherently increase the potential for intraoperative and postoperative hemorrhage. They are indicated for treatment and risk reduction for coronary artery disease (CAD), atrial fibrillation (AF), mechanical heart valves, and deep vein thrombosis (DVT). Because of the underlying diseases, discontinuation of anticoagulant/antiplatelet medications in these patients is not without risk.

The management of hemorrhoids in patients on medications altering coagulation requires careful clinical decision making. Strategies must account for the severity of hemorrhoidal disease, the severity of medical conditions, and the risk related to the (dis)continuation of medications. Literature specifically addressing hemorrhoidal therapy in patients on coagulation-altering drugs is lacking. Therefore, it is important to understand the concepts of management and tailor the approach to the patient. Due to the complexity of some medical conditions, communication with primary care physicians and cardiologists is critical to insure appropriate management.

The purpose of this chapter is to discuss the issues involved with the management of patients with hemorrhoidal disease who are taking medications that alter coagulation. Bleeding risks related to specific hemorrhoidal treatment modalities are addressed. Next, the mechanisms of action of the medications are reviewed. Their use for the treatment of specific conditions and the effects of cessation of use are addressed. Finally, we will propose recommendations addressing the optimal management of patients with symptomatic hemorrhoids taking medications altering coagulation.

Risk of Bleeding with Treatment of Hemorrhoids

A spectrum of therapies has been developed to address symptomatic hemorrhoids. The simplest measures include the addition of fiber to diet and limiting the patient's time on the toilet. Prolonged sitting on the toilet and straining are felt to be associated with hemorrhoidal engorgement and worsening of symptoms. Dietary and behavioral management remain effective strategies for simple hemorrhoidal disease. Alonso-Coello performed a meta-analysis of the utilization of laxatives or fiber

I. Khubchandani et al. (eds.), *Surgical Treatment of Hemorrhoids*, DOI 10.1007/978-1-84800-314-9_28,
© Springer-Verlag London Limited 2009

for patients with hemorrhoids [1]. Fiber supplementation decreased the risk of having persistent symptoms by 53 percent. The risk for continuing bleeding decreased by 50 percent, but improvement in other symptoms did not reach statistical significance. Since these modalities are very low-risk, they have remained the cornerstone of initial treatment.

A number of office procedures have been developed to treat symptomatic early hemorrhoids. These include rubber band ligation (RBL), sclerotherapy, infrared coagulation (IRC), and hemorrhoid artery ligation (HAL). For more advanced hemorrhoids, surgical techniques include the open and closed hemorrhoidectomy and the procedure for prolapse and hemorrhoids (PPH). These modalities have been discussed in detail elsewhere in this text.

A review of the literature reveals a wide range of bleeding rates for these procedures in patients with normal coagulation. Because of heterogeneity in the definition of bleeding, the lack of uniform reporting of the frequency of bleeding requiring directed therapy, and reporting bias, the true incidence of clinically significant bleeding following these procedures is unclear. Reported rates are listed in Table 28.1. The reported incidence of minor bleeding ranges from 0 to 13.6 percent. However, the rate of bleeding requiring operative therapy for control ranges from 0 to 3.0 percent.

Table 28.1 Total and reoperative bleeding rates for hemorrhoid treatment modalities

	Total Bleeding Rate (%)	Reoperative Bleeding Rate
RBL [26, 27, 28, 29]	14/806 (1.7)	6/697 (0.9)
IRC [28, 30, 31, 32]	20/147 (13.6)	0/220 (0)
Sclerotherapy [30, 33, 34]	0/80 (0)	0/201 (0)
Bipolar diathermy [31, 35]	0/75 (0)	0/75 (0)
HAL [36, 37, 38, 39, 40]	21/379 (5.3)	0/274 (0)
PPH [2, 3, 41, 42, 43, 44, 45, 46, 47]	172/4063 (4.2)	108/4767 (2.3)
Harmonic scalpel [48, 49, 50]	1/38 (2.6)	4/538 (0.7)
Milligan-Morgan [2, 42, 43, 47, 49, 50, 51, 52]	15/766 (2.0)	8/816 (1.0)
Ferguson [3, 29, 37, 45, 51, 53, 54]	14/295 (4.7)	9/302 (3.0)

RBL: rubber band ligation; IRC: infrared coagulation; HAL: hemorrhoidal artery ligation; PPH: procedure for prolapse and hemorrhoids

More invasive techniques that transect and ligate the hemorrhoidal vessels (open and closed hemorrhoidectomy and PPH) have the highest rate of operative bleeding.

Different theories exist about the etiology of bleeding following treatment of hemorrhoids. After RBL, sclerotherapy, and IRC, the cause for bleeding is presumed to be ulceration or sloughing of tissue. The time from ligation or IRC to bleeding is usually between 5 and 14 days. Typically, the bleeding that occurs is minor. The incidence of major bleeding requiring surgical therapy or other treatment is small in patients with an intact coagulation mechanism. However, medications that alter coagulation may exacerbate this minor bleeding.

Surgical hemorrhoidectomy carries a higher risk of both minor and clinically significant bleeding. While immediate bleeding after surgery is often related to technical error, late bleeding typically occurs from 5 to 14 days after surgery. The primary theories regarding the etiology of late bleeding following open or closed hemorrhoidectomy postulate local sepsis at the vascular pedicle, which ultimately sloughs, or dissolution of absorbable sutures before vascular healing is complete. There is insufficient evidence to support the use of prophylactic antibiotics to prevent sepsis at the vascular pedicle. Whereas this bleeding is usually self-limited, patients taking anticoagulants may be at higher risk of significant bleeding. Finally, the newer generation of PPH staplers (with a shorter stapling height) are reported to carry a bleeding risk that is slightly less than that following open or closed hemorrhoidectomy [2, 3]. Hemorrhage noted with this technique often occurs in the immediate postoperative period, is profuse, and requires operative placement of a suture ligature. Although there are currently no data to support specific maneuvers to decrease bleeding rates after PPH, some have recommended routine oversewing of the staple line, use of an inflated urinary catheter to tamponade the staple line immediately postoperatively, or overnight observation following treatment for individuals at high risk for bleeding. Since no literature exists at this time, no specific recommendations regarding these approaches can be made.

There is a paucity of literature regarding the treatment of anorectal disease in patients who are taking medications that alter coagulation. A single small case series addresses the use of the LigaSure™ for hemorrhoidectomy in three patients on warfarin [4]. No systematic studies have been done. Traditionally, all anticoagulant or antiplatelet therapy is held preoperatively to minimize the risk of massive bleeding. However, a growing body of medical literature examines the nonsurgical risks related to cessation of these medications, resulting in recommendations that warn against routine discontinuation of medications that alter coagulation.

Medications Altering Coagulation

ASA/NSAIDs

Normal platelet function is a critical component of the coagulation process. Platelets contain a limited amount of the enzyme cyclo-oxygenase type 2 (COX-2), which produces the platelet-activating compound thromboxane A2 (TxA2). Due to platelets' inability to create new proteins, inactivation of COX-2 eliminates the platelets' ability to produce TxA2 [5]. Aspirin irreversibly inactivates COX-2. Therefore, new platelets must be created with active COX-2 to replace those affected by aspirin, a process that requires 7–10 days. In contrast, other NSAIDs reversibly inhibit COX-2. These effects on COX-2 typically resolve in less than 24 h. Although the antiplatelet effects of aspirin may not be reversible, significant bleeding may be controlled with platelet transfusion [5].

Thienopyridines

Thienopyridines are a newer group of medications that affect platelet function. This class of drugs includes clopidogrel (Plavix™) and ticlopidine (Ticlid™). Thienopyridines prevent platelet aggregation by inhibiting the ADP-mediated G-protein activation of cyclic-AMP. In addition, clopidogrel also blocks the binding of fibrinogen to its platelet surface receptor GPIIb/IIIa [5]. Since thienopyridines do not affect COX-1, which produces prostaglandins important for gastric mucosal resistance to acid, they are not directly related to gastrointestinal bleeding [5]. The antiplatelet effects of thienopyridines also cannot directly be reversed, but may be treated with platelet transfusion for severe hemorrhage [5].

Heparin

Heparin/heparinoid medications directly affect components of the coagulation cascade. Specifically, heparin inhibits the function of the activated factors II (thrombin), X, IX, XI and XII [5]. This occurs through heparin's activation of antithrombin III. As this interaction requires only a small component of the heparin molecule, low molecular weight heparins (LMWH) have been developed, which provide a more predictable dose response than unfractionated heparin (UFH). As UFH and LMWH can only be administered parenterally, their utilization is limited to in-hospital and short-term outpatient use. The effect of heparin on coagulation is monitored with the partial thromboplastin time (PTT). Although monitoring the effects of LMWH are not usually necessary, it may be advisable in some patient populations, including the morbidly obese and patients with renal failure [5]. The College of American Pathologists recommends the anti-Xa assay, as high circulating levels of anti-Xa are associated with clinical bleeding. The effects of heparin may be neutralized with protamine, using a ratio of 1 mg of protamine per 100 U of unfractionated heparin [5].

Warfarin

Warfarin directly affects the components of the extrinsic clotting cascade. Specifically, it interferes with the vitamin K-mediated carboxylation of factors II, VII, IX, and X [5]. The main suppression of coagulation results primarily from its effect on factor II (prothrombin). In addition, warfarin also inhibits the carboxylation of the anticoagulant factors, protein C and protein S. This inhibition of the anticoagulant factors occurs first, as they have a shorter biological half-life than the procoagulant clotting factors, resulting in a transient hypercoagulable state. Monitoring of the effects of warfarin on coagulation is done by the prothrombin time (PT) and the international normalized ratio (INR). The effects of warfarin on coagulation may be reversed by the administration of vitamin K or the administration of fresh frozen plasma to restore the PT to near normal levels.

Nutritional Supplements

Use of herbal therapies for a variety of conditions is very common. It has been recognized that a number of these agents may in fact increase the risk of bleeding, both by altering the metabolism or binding of antiplatelet and anticoagulant medications, or by direct effects on the clotting cascade. Herbal supplements known to possess antiplatelet activity include bilberry, dong quai, feverfew, garlic, ginger, ginko, ginseng, meadowsweet, turmeric, and willow. Herbs that contain coumarin include chamomile, fenugreek, horse chestnut, motherwort, red clover, and tamarind. As these nutraceuticals are not critical medications taken for diseases to be discussed below, the literature currently recommends stopping these supplements 1–2 weeks prior to surgery [6].

Hemorrhoidal Therapy in Patients with Altered Coagulation

General Considerations

In all of these patients, the first decision that has to be made concerns the severity of the hemorrhoidal symptoms and the need for surgical or nonsurgical intervention. We must follow the rule "to do no harm." Fortunately, hemorrhoidal disease is rarely life threatening. Therapy in these patients should not be undertaken without thorough discussion and clear informed consent regarding the risks and benefits of various treatments. Occasionally, patients on coagulation-altering medications will

have hemorrhoidal bleeding sufficient to require repeated transfusions. In other patients, chronic prolapse with seepage and mucous secretion may produce an intolerable situation.

In general, we avoid sequential single quadrant rubber band ligation, a technique that we commonly use in patients with intact coagulation. We would, instead, favor surgical excision of the hemorrhoids with careful pedicle ligation and closure of the wounds with a slowly absorbed suture such as polyglactin 910 (Vicryl™). We believe such a technique will lower the risk of postoperative bleeding in the 5–14 days after surgery. If band ligation is to be considered, it seems reasonable to ligate all symptomatic hemorrhoids at one time rather than exposing the patient to repeated episodes of risk from withdrawal of the anticoagulants.

Specific Medical Conditions

Hemorrhoid Therapy in Patients with CAD and Coronary Stents

Coronary artery disease (CAD) is a very common condition, which encompasses angina, previous myocardial infarction (MI), and previous coronary artery bypass graft (CABG). Commonly, lifelong aspirin use is recommended, with thienopyridine medications used as an adjunct to coronary arterial patency. Discontinuation of aspirin is noted to carry greater than a 3-fold increase in major cardiac adverse events at a mean time of 10 days [7].

The use of coronary stents has revolutionized the management of CAD. Placement of stents contributes to better long-term patency rates and delays restenosis of the coronary vessels. Despite these long-term improvements in coronary artery patency, stent placement does carry the short-term risk of stent thrombosis. This is related to denuding of the vascular endothelium, which requires approximately eight weeks to re-endothelialize. This process is platelet-mediated, making antiplatelet medications essential for prevention. Multivariate analysis has identified antiplatelet medication cessation as a major predictor of stent occlusion [8, 9]. The cardiac risk associated with noncardiac surgery early following stent placement is particularly high. This risk is greatest during the first six weeks following percutaneous coronary intervention [10].

For these reasons, the ACC/AHA has made a number of recommendations for perioperative management of patients with coronary stents. First, cardiology consultation is necessary prior to discontinuation of any antiplatelet agent before surgery. If possible, elective surgery with a risk of bleeding that necessitates discontinuation of antiplatelet agents should be deferred at least one month for patients with bare metal stent (BMS) and 12 months for those with drug eluting stent (DES). Finally, aspirin should be continued throughout the procedure with resumption of thienopyridine medications postoperatively as soon as possible, potentially within a few days [11].

The decision whether to continue antiplatelet medications perioperatively balances the surgical bleeding risks against potential cardiac events. Hemorrhoid therapy differs from most general surgical procedures in that it carries a risk of major and minor bleeding which is remote from the time of treatment. For this reason, recommendations applicable to general surgical procedures to withhold medications perioperatively may not be appropriate if extended for the entire period of risk for hemorrhoid surgery.

Because of the concerns about thrombosis, a growing body of literature has evaluated the continued use of anticoagulant and antiplatelet medications during the perioperative period. However, there is limited evidence specific to general surgery or anorectal surgery. The American Society of Gastroenterology (ASGE) has published guidelines which address the use of anticoagulant/antiplatelet medications during endoscopic procedures [12, 13]. Generally, in low risk procedures (e.g., colonoscopy with cold biopsy), anticoagulant/antiplatelet medications (including warfarin, aspirin, NSAIDs, and thienopyridine medications) are considered safe; however, snare polypectomy is considered a high risk procedure for which anticoagulation and antiplatelet agents should be held. The physician must assess the inherent risk of thromboembolic complications versus bleeding risk to manage such patients. The risk for late bleeding after snare polypectomy is probably similar to that following hemorrhoidal therapy. The current literature indicates there is limited risk of significant bleeding following minor surgery if the patient is taking aspirin or NSAIDs [9, 14, 15, 16]. More limited information is present for thienopyridines. Both aspirin and thienopyridines function as antiplatelet agents. However, in the experience of the authors, thienopyridine medications appear to have more potent effects, leading to troublesome bleeding postoperatively.

Due to the cardiac risk related to cessation of aspirin and thienopyridine medications in patients with CAD or previous coronary stent placement, patients may benefit from continuing these medications during the perioperative period. If a patient is on both types of medication, consultation with the cardiologist will be necessary to determine if a single medication is sufficient during the perioperative period. Since the time to reverse the effects of both aspirin and thienopyridine medications is 7–10 days, to avoid the bleeding risk of dual drug coverage, one medication (preferably the thienopyridine) would be withheld for a total of 2–3 weeks (one week preoperatively, 1–2 weeks postoperatively). Utilization of a bridging strategy during cessation of antiplatelet agents may be considered. However, since coronary artery and stent thrombosis is a platelet-mediated phenomenon, heparin/LMWH may not offer adequate phophylaxis. In this setting, shorter-acting medications such as non-aspirin NSAIDs may be considered. The effectiveness of this strategy, however, is unclear. It must be noted that thrombosis typically occurs during or after surgery [14].

For lower grade hemorrhoids, dietary and behavioral modification would be appropriate as an initial treatment. Less invasive measures may be utilized, including IRC, RBL, sclerotherapy, and HAL. One of our colleagues, in an unreported series, has performed more than 300 ligations on patients taking aspirin with but a single episode of bleeding. He injects the base and the ligated areas with sodium morrhuate. The risk of major bleeding associated with these treatment modalities is low, but unpredictable in patients on antiplatelet agents. However, the patient must be informed of the potential risk for major bleeding in the first two weeks postoperatively. Furthermore, the patient should be educated regarding the expected amount of minor bleeding. It may be advisable to suggest that the patient remain in close proximity to the surgeon for at least 14 days after the procedure in case major bleeding does occur.

For patients with a significant external component, advanced grade 3 or grade 4 disease, a more invasive approach may be necessary. The newer model of the PPH stapler has a lower reported rate of significant bleeding. Selected patients with grade 3 disease may be treated with this method if a meticulous technique is used to ensure no bleeding from the staple line; however, no prospective evidence exists regarding its use in patients taking antiplatelet medications. Both open and closed hemorrhoidectomy carry a higher risk of late major bleeding. However, these approaches may be necessary for patients with a major external component or grade 4 internal and external hemorrhoids. In all patients with altered coagulation states, regardless of the agent used, one may consider placement of an additional suture ligature at the apex of the hemorrhoidectomy site to decrease the risk of secondary hemorrhage. Another consideration is to use a more slowly absorbable suture such as polyglactin 910 (Vicryl^{TM}) for wound closure. In the experience of the authors, if excisional treatment can be limited to the quadrant or quadrants with the most severe disease, suture ligation (or Doppler-guided HAL) may be used as an adjunct in areas of lesser disease in order to decrease bleeding risk. Again, however, no good evidence has been published to specifically address this issue.

Hemorrhoid Therapy in Patients with AF

Atrial fibrillation (AF) is a recognized risk factor for the development of arterial embolic disease, leading to stroke or other arterial occlusion. Therefore, patients with AF are frequently maintained on long-term warfarin therapy. Utilization of warfarin decreases the risk of stroke by 66–80 percent [17, 18]. Less commonly, patients may receive aspirin therapy instead, which produces a 50–80 percent risk reduction in lower risk patients [19].

Studies have evaluated the additional risk related to patients with AF who stop their medical therapy for short durations of time, as for surgery. Patients with AF and without previous stroke have

a perioperative stroke incidence of 0.08–0.2 percent, compared to 2.1–2.9 percent stroke risk if the patient has had a previous stroke [17, 18, 20]. The mean interval from aspirin discontinuation to stroke in at-risk patients was 9.5 days [21].

A number of risk factors have been identified for perioperative stroke and thromboembolism in patients with AF. These risk factors include age greater than 75, a history of diabetes, hypertension, previous transient ischemic attack or stroke, and left ventricular dysfunction [18]. Patients with AF complicated by one or more of these risk factors may benefit from heparin bridging. Bridging usually involves administration of heparin or LWMH by injection during the time when the warfarin levels are nontherapeutic, withholding heparin the day of surgery, and resuming heparin or LMWH postoperatively until warfarin treatment results in an appropriate INR. However, patients without risk factors do not have a sufficient risk to merit a bridging strategy. Traditionally, an INR of 1.4 has been used as "safe" in terms of bleeding risk.

Dunn performed a systematic review of the hemorrhagic and thromboembolic risk associated with different warfarin management protocols [22]. This review concluded that oral anticoagulants could be continued during minor procedures (dental extractions, joint and soft tissue injections, cataract surgery, upper and lower endoscopy with biopsy) without major bleeding risk. However, use of warfarin during major surgery carried a prohibitive risk of major bleeding. Therefore, cessation of warfarin with or without heparin bridging was recommended. Ultimately, the decision in the context of this chapter lies in whether one considers hemorrhoid treatment to be a major or minor procedure. (With regard to bleeding risk, the senior author, HRB, considers it to be a major procedure.) As indicated previously, major bleeding following hemorrhoidectomy occurs when most patients would be fully anticoagulated, regardless of the perioperative anticoagulation management. One of the authors, HRB, discontinues warfarin on the day of RBL and resumes anticoagulation 10 days after RBL. This strategy ensures a window between the 5th and 14th day after surgery when the patient is not fully anticoagulated. Further study is necessary to determine the optimal periprocedural strategy.

Patients at high risk for thromboembolic disease would likely benefit from a bridging protocol. The risk for major bleeding complications postoperatively persists, however. Recommendations for the patient to remain close to medical services may be appropriate. Short-term transition from warfarin to an antiplatelet agent may serve as an intermediate level of coverage to limit thromboembolic and bleeding risk; however, further study is needed.

For lower-grade hemorrhoids, dietary and behavioral modification is appropriate as an initial step. It is unclear whether RBL and IRC carry a prohibitive bleeding risk in this patient population. Techniques with a lower bleeding risk may be considered, such as sclerotherapy or HAL. However, prospective data in studies large enough to have statistical power to differentiate between these techniques are lacking.

More severe grade-3 or grade-4 hemorrhoids, or those with a significant external component, may require a surgical approach. Patients with AF and no additional risk factors may be adequately treated with warfarin cessation and surgery, with return to warfarin therapy 10 days postoperatively. Studies do not elucidate the specific risk related to oral anticoagulation following hemorrhoidectomy. Rosen reported a 0.8 percent incidence of bleeding following hemorrhoidectomy. The median time to bleeding in his series was six days postoperatively [23]. Of the patients who required directed therapy, 22 percent were using antiplatelet agents and 15 percent were using warfarin. It is unclear what proportion of all patients taking an anticoagulant or antiplatelet agent that these figures represent. The decision regarding whether to discontinue warfarin and whether to use a bridging strategy will depend upon the surgeon's and medical doctor's comfort. Further study is needed to clarify this issue.

Hemorrhoid Therapy in Patients with Mechanical Heart Valves

Patients who have had mechanical heart valve placement are at a significant risk of thromboembolic complications. The reported rate without anticoagulation is four percent per year. The risk is highest for patients with caged ball valves, mechanical mitral valves, atrial fibrillation, previous thromboembolism, left ventricular dysfunction, and hypercoagulable states [24, 25]. Warfarin-based anticoagulation reduces the risk of thromboembolic complications by 75 percent.

Based upon the available data, the ACC and AHA produced guidelines for the management of anticoagulants perioperatively in patients with mechanical heart valves [24]. For patients with a low risk of thromboembolism (aortic valves with no risk factors, as above), warfarin may be discontinued 48–72 h preoperatively and be resumed 24 h postoperatively, without the need for bridging. For patients at high risk of thromboembolism (aortic valves with risk factors or mitral valves), bridging therapy with UFH or LMWH may be used.

The above recommendation needs to be tailored to the risk of hemorrhoid surgery. In the authors' opinions, this minor surgery carries a significant risk of major bleeding if the patient is fully anticoagulated during the 5–14 day postoperative window. Although antiplatelet agents are reported to decrease the risk of thromboembolic complications 45 percent (versus 75 percent with warfarin), their use is not currently supported as an alternative to anticoagulation [25].

The surgical recommendations for treating hemorrhoidal disease are similar to those for patients on chronic warfarin for AF. The importance of meticulous surgical technique cannot be understated. Also, it is important to consult with the patient's cardiologist to utilize the appropriate anticoagulation strategy.

Hemorrhoid Therapy in Patients with DVT

Deep vein thrombosis (DVT) is a relatively common condition that often requires anticoagulation therapy. In sporadic cases of DVT, warfarin therapy is typically recommended for six months. However, some patients with hypercoagulable states or recurrent DVT may require lifelong therapy. In contrast to arterial thromboembolic disease, surgery has been found to increase the risk of DVT and venous thromboembolism. This is particularly important in patients with previous DVT, in which 6 percent of recurrent DVT are fatal [17]. The initial period after developing a DVT carries the greatest risk of embolic disease, approaching 40 percent during the first month, 10 percent during the second and third months, and 15 percent annually, thereafter [17, 18].

Hemorrhoids rarely require emergency surgery. Therefore it is reasonable to wait for at least three months after the development of DVT so that aggressive anticoagulation can be pursued during this critical period. After this time, warfarin can be stopped and surgery may proceed, most often with a bridging strategy. After six months warfarin may be stopped and surgery can proceed in the usual fashion.

Although office-based procedures likely do not carry the risk of recurrent DVT that would be expected with surgery under general or spinal anesthesia, treatment of a fully anticoagulated patient may place the patient at higher risk of bleeding complications.

Less common is the person who requires life-long anticoagulation for recurrent DVT secondary to a hypercoagulable state. In such situations, communication with the primary care physician or hematologist may be necessary to ensure appropriate periprocedural anticoagulant management. Depending upon the patient risk for recurrent venous thromboembolic disease, a heparin/LMWH bridging strategy may be appropriate. The general treatment approach would be similar to patients requiring warfarin therapy for other conditions. Again, we emphasize that meticulous surgical technique is essential to minimize hemorrhagic complications.

Other Conditions

There are a number of other medical conditions for which patients take medications that alter coagulation. The most common of these is NSAID use for arthritic or other pain. Although the current evidence indicates limited risk related to continuation of aspirin and NSAIDs during minor surgery, it is the opinion of the authors that these medications should be withheld during the duration of treatment. Since these medications are being taken for

conditions that are not life threatening, it would be prudent to limit the potential for adverse effects as much as possible.

Conclusions

Symptomatic hemorrhoids are common and affect all segments of the population. An increasing number of patients are on medications that alter coagulation and it is not uncommon to come across a patient with symptomatic hemorrhoids who is on these medications. The additional surgical and medical risk related to the continuation or discontinuation of antiplatelet or anticoagulant medications is important to recognize. As our understanding of these thromboembolic risks improves, the surgical paradigm may shift to permit a broader number of procedures to be performed while the patient is under the effects of antiplatelet or anticoagulant medications. It is clear that further study needs to be done to elucidate this issue in anorectal surgery. Due to the paucity or absence of data supporting many of our recommendations, we would favor assembling a panel of "experts" to formulate a consensus or "best practices" on these management issues.

References

1. Alonso-Coello P, Guyatt G, Heels-Ansell D, Johanson J, Lopez-Yarto M, Mills E, Zhou Q. Laxatives for the treatment of hemorrhoids. Cochrane Database Syst Rev 2005, Issue 4. Art. No.: CD004649. DOI: 10.1002/14651858. CD004649.pub2
2. Ortiz H, Marzo J, Armendariz P. Randomized clinical trial of stapled haemorrhoidopexy versus conventional diathermy haemorrhoidectomy. Br J Surg 2002;89:1376–1381
3. Senagore A, Singer M, Abcarian H, Fleshman J, Corman M, Wexner S, Nivatvongs S. A prospective, randomized, controlled multicenter trial comparing stapled hemorrhoidopexy and Ferguson hemorrhoidectomy: perioperative and one-year results. Dis Colon Rectum 2004;47
4. Lawes D, Palazzo F, Clifton M. The use of LigaSure™ haemorrhoidectomy in patients taking oral anticoagulation therapy. Colorectal Dis 2004;6:111–112
5. Owens C, Belkin M. Thrombosis and coagulation: operative management of the anticoagulated patient. Surg Clin N Am 2005;85:1179–1189

6. Ang-Lee M, Moss J, Yuan C. Herbal medicines and perioperative care. JAMA 2001;286:208–216

7. Biondi-Zoccai G, Lotrionte M, Agostoni P, Abbate A, Fusaro M, Burzotta F, Testa L, Sheiban I, Sangiorgi G. A systematic review and meta-analysis on the hazards of discontinuing or not adhering to aspirin among 50,279 patients at risk for coronary artery disease. Eur Heart J 2006;27:2667–2674

8. Ferrari E, Benhamou M, Cerboni P, Marcel B. Coronary syndromes following aspirin withdrawal: a special risk for late stent thrombosis. J Am Coll Cardiol 2005;45:456–459

9. Spahn D, Howell S, Delabays A, Chassot P. Coronary stents and perioperative anti-platelet regimen: dilemma of bleeding and stent thrombosis. Br J Anaesth 2006;96: 675–7

10. Mendoza C, Virani S, Shah N, Ferreira A, Marchena E. Noncardiac surgery following percutaneous coronary intervention. Catheter Cardiovasc Interv 2004;63:267–273

11. Grines C, Bonow R, Casey J, Gardner T, Lockhart P, Moliterno D, O'Gara P, Whitlow P. Prevention of premature discontinuation of dual antiplatelet therapy in patients with coronary artery stents: a science advisory from the American Heart Association, American College of Cardiology, Society for Cardiovascular Angiography and Interventions, American College of Surgeons, and American Dental Association, with representation from the American College of Physicians. J Am Coll Cardiol 2007;49:734–739

12. Eisen G, Baron T, Dominitz J, Faigel D, Goldstein J, Johanson J, Mallery J, Raddawi H, Vargo J, Waring J. Guideline on the management of anticoagulation and antiplatelet therapy for endoscopic procedures. Gastrointest Endosc 2002;55:775–779

13. Zuckerman M, Hirota W, Adler D, Davila R, Jacobson B, Leighton J, Qureshi W, Rajan E, Hambrick R, Fanelli R, Baron T, Faigel D. ASGE guideline: The management of low-molecular-weight heparin and nonaspirin antiplatelet agents for endoscopic procedures. Gastrointest Endosc 2005;61:189–194

14. Brilakis E, Banerjee S, Berger P. Perioperative management of patients with coronary stents. J Am Coll Cardiol 2007; 49:2145–2150

15. Cardwell M, Siviter G, Smith A. Nonsteroidal anti-inflammatory drugs and perioperative bleeding in paediatric tonsillectomy. Cochrane Database Syst Rev 2005, Issue 2. Art. No.: CD003591. DOI: 10.1002/14651858.CD003591.pub2

16. Shalom A, Wong L. Outcome of aspirin use during excision of cutaneous lesions. Ann Plast Surg 2003;50:296–298

17. Kearon C, Hirsh J. Management of anticoagulation before and after elective surgery. N Engl J Med 1997;336: 1506–1511

18. Spyopoulos A, Turpie A. Perioperative bridging interruption with heparin for the patient receiving long-term anticoagulation. Curr Opin Intern Med 2005;4:602–608

19. Stroke Prevention in Atrial Fibrillation I Trial. Warfarin versus aspirin for prevention of thromboembolism in atrial fibrillation: Stroke Prevention in Atrial Fibrillation II Study. Lancet 1994;343:687–691

20. Vink R, Rienstra M, van Dongen C, Levi M, Buller H, Crijns H, van Gelder I. Risk of thromboembolism and bleeding after general surgery in patients with atrial fibrillation. Am J Cardiol 2005;96:822–824

21. Maulaz A, Bezerra D, Michel P, Bogousslavsky J. Effect of discontinuing aspirin therapy on the risk of brain ischemic stroke. Arch Neurol 2005;62:1217–1220

22. Dunn A, Turpie A. Perioperative management of patients receiving oral anticoagulants: a systematic review. Arch Intern Med 2003;163:901–908

23. Rosen L, Sipe P, Stasik J, Riether R, Trimpi H. Outcome of delayed hemorrhage following surgical hemorrhoidectomy. Dis Colon Rectum 1993;36:743–746

24. Bonow R, Carabello B, Chatterjee K, de Leon A, Jr., Faxon D, Freed M, Gaasch W, Lytle B, Nishimura R, O'Gara P, O'Rourke R, Otto C, Shah P, Shanewise J, Smith S Jr, Jacobs A, Adams C, Anderson J, Antman E, Faxon D, Fuster V, Halperin J, Hiratzka L, Hunt S, Lytle B, Nishimura R, Page R, Riegel B. ACC/AHA 2006 practice guidelines for the management of patients with valvular heart disease: executive summary: a report of the American College of Cardiology/American Heart Association Task Force on Practice Guidelines (writing committee to revise the 1998 guidelines for the management of patients with valvular heart disease) developed in collaboration with the Society of Cardiovascular Anesthesiologists endorsed by the Society for Cardiovascular Angiography and Interventions and the Society of Thoracic Surgeons. J Am Coll Cardiol 2006;48:598–675

25. Cannegieter S, Rosendaal F, Briet E. Thromboembolic and bleeding complications in patients with mechanical heart valve prostheses. Circulation 1994;89:635–641

26. Armstrong D. Multiple hemorrhoidal ligation: a prospective, randomized trial evaluating a new technique. Dis Colon Rectum 2003;46:179–186

27. Bat L, Melzer E, Koler M, Dreznick Z, Shemesh E. Complications of rubber band ligation of symptomatic internal hemorrhoids. Dis Colon Rectum 1993;36:287–290

28. Gupta P. Infrared coagulation versus rubber band ligation in early stage hemorrhoids. Braz J Med Biol Res 2003;36: 1433–1439

29. Shanmugam V, Thaha M, Rabindranath K, Campbell K, Steele R, Loudon M. Systematic review of randomized trials comparing rubber band ligation with excisional haemorrhoidectomy. Br J Surg 2005;92

30. Ambrose N, Morris D, Alexander-Williams J, Keighley M. A randomized trial of photocoagulation or injection sclerotherapy for the treatment of first- and second-degree hemorrhoids. Dis Colon Rectum 1985;28

31. Dennison A, Whiston R, Rooney S, Chadderton R, Wherry D, Morris D. A randomized comparison of infrared photocoagulation with bipolar diathermy for the outpatient treatment of hemorrhoids. Dis Colon Rectum 1990;33: 32–34

32. Leicester R, Nicholls R, Mann C. Infrared coagulation: a new treatment for hemorrhoids. Dis Colon Rectum 1981; 24:602–605

33. Jaspersen D. Doppler sonographic diagnostic and treatment control of symptomatic first-degree hemorrhoids: preliminary report and results. Dig Dis Sci 1993;38

34. Kanellos I, Goulimaris I, Christoforidis E, Kelpis T, Betsis D. A comparison of the simultaneous application of sclerotherapy and rubber band ligation, with sclerotherapy and rubber band ligation applied separately, for the treatment of haemorrhoids: a prospective randomized trial. Colorectal Dis 2003;5:133–138

35. Hinton C, Morris D. A randomized trial comparing direct current therapy and bipolar diathermy in the outpatient treatment of third-degree hemorrhoids. Dis Colon Rectum 1992;33:931–932

36. Arnold S, Antonietti E, Rollinger G, Scheyer M. Doppler-sonographisch unterstutzte hamorrhoiden-arterienligatur. Chirurg 2002;73:269–273

37. Bursics A, Morvay K, Kupcsulik P, Flautner L. Comparison of early and 1-year follow-up results of conventional hemorrhoidectomy and hemorrhoid artery ligation: a randomized study. Int J Colorectal Dis 2004;19:176–180

38. Felice G, Privitera A, Ellul E, Klaumann M. Doppler-guided hemorrhoidal artery ligation: an alternative to hemorrhoidectomy. Dis Colon Rectum 2005;48

39. Morinaga K, Hasuda K, Ikeda T. A novel therapy for internal hemorrhoids: ligation of the hemorrhoidal artery with a newly devised instrument (Moricorn) in conjunction with a Doppler flowmeter. Am J Gastroenterol 1995; 90:610–613

40. Sohn N, Aronoff J, Cohen F, Weinstein M. Transanal hemorrhoidal dearterialization is an alternative to operative hemorrhoidectomy. Am J Surg 2001;182:515–519

41. Arroyo A, Perez-Vicente F, Miranda E, Sanchez A, Serrano P, Candela F, Oliver I, Calpena R. Prospective randomized clinical trial comparing two different circular staplers for mucosectomy in the treatment of hemorrhoids. World J Surg 2006;30:1305–1310

42. Ganio E, Altomare D, Gabrielli F, Milito G, Canuti S. Prospective randomized multicentre trial comparing stapled with open haemorrhoidectomy. Br J Surg 2001; 88:669–674

43. Gravie J, Lehur P, Huten N, Papillon M, Fantoli M, Descottes B, Pessaux P, Arnaud J. Stapled hemorrhoidopexy versus Milligan-Morgan hemorrhoidectomy: a prospective, randomized, multicenter trial with 2-year postoperative follow up. Ann Surg 2005;242:29–35

44. Jongen J, Bock J, Peleikis H, Eberstein A, Pfister K. Complications and reoperations in stapled anopexy: learning by doing. Int J Colorectal Dis 2006;21:166–171

45. Kraemer M, Parulava T, Roblick M, Duschka L, Muller-Lobeck H. Prospective, randomized study: proximate PPH stapler vs. LigaSure for hemorrhoidal surgery. Dis Colon Rectum 2005;48:1517–1522

46. Ng K, Ho K, Ooi B, Tang C, Eu K. Experience of 3711 stapled haemorrhoidectomy operations. Br J Surg 2006;93: 226–230

47. Shalaby R, Desoky A. Randomized clinical trial of stapled versus Milligan-Morgan haemorrhoidectomy. Br J Surg 2001;88:1049–1053

48. Armstrong D, Frankum C, Schertzer M, Ambroze W, Orangio G. Harmonic scalpel hemorrhoidectomy. Dis Colon Rectum 2002;45:354–359

49. Jayne D, Botterill I, Ambrose N, Brennan T, Guillou P, O'Riordain D. Randomized clinical trial of LigaSure™ versus conventional diathermy for day-case haemorrhoidectomy. Br J Surg 2002;89

50. Palazzo F, Francis D, Clifton M. Randomized clinical trial of LigaSure™ versus open haemorrhoidectomy. Br J Surg 2002;89:154–157

51. Arbman G, Krook H, Haapaniemi S. Closed vs. open hemorrhoidectomy—is there any difference? Dis Colon Rectum 2000;43:31–34

52. Sayfan J. Complications of Milligan-Morgan hemorrhoidectomy. Dig Surg 2001;18:131–133

53. Bleday R, Pena J, Rothenberger D, Goldberg S, Buls J. Symptomatic hemorrhoids: current incidence and complications of operative therapy. Dis Colon Rectum 1992;35: 477–481

54. Khalil K, O'Bichere A, Sellu D. Randomized clinical trial of sutured versus stapled closed haemorrhoidectomy. Br J Surg 2000;87:1352–1355

Landmarks in the History of Hemorrhoids

Charles V. Mann

Date	Comments
c. 2250 BC	Code of Hammurabi, King of Babylon. Description of anal symptoms (hemorrhoids).
1700 BC	Edwin Smith papyrus. Use of astringent lotions for anal symptoms (hemorrhoids?) described.
1552 BC	Eber papyrus. The most complete record of Egyptian medicine. Hemorrhoid remedies described.
460–375 BC	Writings of Hippocrates. Treatment of hemorrhoids by cautery and excision described.
Old Testament, Samuel 5:9	Philistines punished with "emerods."
Old Testament Samuel 5:12	After the Ark moved to Ekron, perpetrators smitten by "emerods."
25 BC–AD 50	Celsus describes ligature of piles with flax.
AD 130–200	Galen recommends conservative management of piles (laxatives, ointments, leeches) and regards bleeding as therapeutic. Also describes, however, use of a tight thread to induce sloughing of hemorrhoids.
Sometime between the fourth & sixth century AD	Susruta Samhita describes use of treatment by clamp and cautery method.
10th century AD	El-Zahrawy describes treatment by application of cautery irons.
10th–15th century AD	Treatment in Byzantine medical practise by twisting pile, application of ligature to its base, followed by amputation—a "modern" approach that lapses for many centuries.
1307–1370	John of Arderne publishes his treatise on the treatment of fistula and hemorrhoids, and the use of clysters (enemas).

Date	Comments
1660–1734	Georg Ernst Stahl publishes a classic work on the treatment of hemorrhoids.
1835	Foundation of St. Marks Hospital, London, by Frederick Salmon for the treatment of anal diseases, especially fistula in ano and hemorrhoids.
1849	J. G. Maisonneuve describes treatment by forceful anal dilation. Subsequently, this treatment is revived by P. H. Lord.
1935	Development of the classical method of open dissection and ligature at St. Marks Hospital by E. T. C. Milligan and C. Naughton Morgan.
1955	Development of a closed method of hemorrhoidectomy by A. G. Parks, London.
1960	The closed surgical method of treatment established by J. A. Ferguson and colleagues at Grand Rapids, Missouri.
1963	Invention of the method of rubber band ligation of hemorrhoids as an office procedure by J. Barron (USA). Method widely adopted thereafter.
1970	New methods for physical destruction of hemorrhoids developed (cryotherapy infrared thermocoagulation, diathermy, laser). Some still used.
1975	Use of anal dilatation advocated by P. H. Lord. Is not widely adopted but of historical importance. Classical studies by W. H. F. Thomson into the nature of hemorrhoids and their development from anal cushions, which are normal structures.
1990	Day-case surgery initiated in special centers.

Index

Printed in the United States of America